MW01178895

PRAISE FOR
THE 7-DAY DIGITAL DIET

"Never has the world needed conscious listening more than now, and never has it been more challenged – largely by our obsession with our devices. Fear of missing out (FOMO) is ironically causing us to miss out, on our key relationships. Our happiness, effectiveness and well-being are being hurt as we to relate more to our phones than to our friends and colleagues. In this superb book, Tim David offers a tonic for the ages: a simple, practical program that rediscovers balance and delivers a healthy human/device relationship so we can get the best out of technology while preserving our human connections. This book is essential for anyone with a phone!"

– Julian Treasure, five-time TED speaker and author of the award-winning book, *How To Be Heard*

"Do you spend more time looking at your phone's screen than at the human beings around you? Tim David's book will engage and amuse you even as it gives you the tools to 'unhook' yourself in just a week."

– Roger Dooley, author of *Friction* and *Brainfluence*

"Technology is a big part of our lives, but it isn't everything. *The 7-Day Digital Diet* keeps the best of technology and removes the worst so you can do more good stuff!"

– Joel Comm, *New York Times* bestselling author

"Tim David's *7-Day Digital Diet* is a down-to-earth (and downright entertaining) manual for navigating smartphone overuse in the 21st Century. David's approach teaches you to extract the benefits of having a smartphone without succumbing to its many costs, and rightly suggests that going cold turkey isn't an option in a world as deeply connected as ours. A must-read if you're one of the millions struggling to get the most from your phone without letting it get the best of you."

– Adam Alter, Professor of Marketing and Psychology, New York University Stern School of Business and *New York Times* bestselling author, *Irresistible* and *Drunk Tank Pink*

"Admitting you've got a digital addiction is the first step. But the remaining steps can be unclear and just as difficult. Luckily, Tim David is here to guide us with a fast and effective recovery plan. Read this book...just don't read it on your phone."

– David Burkus, author of *Pick A Fight*

"In *The 7-Day Digital Diet* Tim David gives practical advice on striking a balance between our offline and online behaviors. What excites me most is that if we all put this into practice the world will be a better place."

– Erik Qualman, #1 Bestselling Author of *Digital Leader*

"In a world where couples are more likely to break up via text than in person, and families go out to dinner to have conversations with their phones and personal devices, Tim David's book offers a refreshing and practical alternative to the challenge of connection in a digital, and often distracting, age. *The 7 Day Digital Diet* is a fun, practical must-read for anyone who wants to be more present, more in control, and more joyful."

– Alan Samuel Cohen, Author of *The Connection Challenge: How Executives Create Power and Possibility in The Age of Distraction*

"Tim has written an important and timely guide to breaking your phone addiction. I skipped right to the chapter for parents, then went back to the beginning for myself. Because even though I wrote a book on how to work with focus, I'm as guilty as everyone else when it comes to getting distracted by technology. This is a digital diet you can actually do and as an added bonus, Tim's writing's funny too."

– Joshua Seth, star of *Digimon* and author of *Finding Focus in a Changing World*

"The customer experience is heavily affected by individual interactions and relationships - the very things we're losing as technology increases. This book will help your employees connect with one another better, connect with customers better, and create a richer customer experience. Highly recommended!"

– Shep Hyken, customer service/experience expert and *New York Times* bestselling author

THE 7-DAY DIGITAL DIET

First published by Tim David 2020

First edition June 2020

Tim David

THE 7-DAY DIGITAL DIET

HOW TO USE YOUR PHONE LESS AND LIVE MORE

TIM DAVID

TABLE OF CONTENTS

Human Connection

Nothing is more
valuable than

my phone

I don’t *need*

face-to-face interaction

I’ve realized I crave

digital consumption

more than

human connection

what matters is

my perspective

versus

your perspective

things are not

how they used to be

I’ve learned that
people aren’t

concerned about
empathy

the average
person is

staring at a screen
for 7 hours a day

the best things
in life aren’t
happening

later...things need
to happen NOW!

we can’t make
change in this
world

FORWARD

I know. I spelled it "Forward," as in, "the opposite of backward." It's supposed to be "Foreword," as in, "a short introductory statement" (and the opposite of "Backeword?")

Don't worry about the spelling. Like performing Shakespeare in a hospital, it was just a play on wards.

The meaning is what matters. The meaning you draw from something is always more important than what that something actually is. Two people can ride the exact same roller coaster and one will feel a rush of excitement and joy while the other feels abject terror. Two people can read the exact same pun and one will laugh out loud while the other feels abject terror.

When you read the preceding pages, you probably understood a message of pessimism and defeat. Let's turn that around. Literally.

Read the same words again, but this time, flip through the pages *BACKWARD*.

Start on the page that says, "we can't make change in this world." Read it. Then, read the page before it. Then continue until you get to the title page, "Human Connection." Do that now and then come back here. (For a video demonstration, visit 7DayDigitalDiet.com/fun.)

The meaning has completely changed, hasn't it?

That's what happens when you look at something with a new perspective.

This book was not written for the Luddite, who believes that we should set off an EMP so large that it renders every device a digital carcass and puts us all back into the Renaissance. It was not written for the mother who put her kids' devices on a stump and shot them with a shotgun (true story.) It's not a technophobic manifesto or a love song to the good old days. But it wasn't written for the guy who married one of his devices either. (You'll read about him later.) This book is not some glorified hardbound permission slip for screens to claim more and more grains of sand from our hourglasses. Neither extreme is practical. Our only hope is if we read the poem in both directions and learn a little something each time.

As a species, we're at an interesting moment in our history—perhaps even a crucial one. Our honeymoon period with the smartphone is over. Sure, we love our smartphone technology and we'd marry it all over again, but we're also learning a lot about our new partner that we don't like. It giveth and it taketh away.

We're faced with a similar conundrum almost every time a new technology shows up. Some people get excited and some people get scared. (Remember the time Socrates complained about those new-fangled things called "books?" Devil's work, those books.) But if there's one thing we can learn from history, it's that technology doesn't move backwards. Phones aren't going anywhere—and we wouldn't really want them to. The question is, can we learn to live with them?

So, who is this book for? It's for the person who feels like they might be on their phone too much. It's for the person who likes their phone, plans on keeping it, but realizes that sometimes it distracts them from what (and who) really matters. Our relationship with technology is flawed but it is here to stay. Let's not fight it. Let's not flee it. Let's diet.

iPEED MYSELF

Yup. We just met and you're already getting the "I peed myself" story.

Now, I don't normally do this.

Trust me, it's not always, "Hi, I'm Tim David and I peed myself a little." I'm not like Forrest Gump in that scene where he meets the President.

But you? I've already told you "I peed myself" three times. Four, if you count the title of this chapter. And we're only on page one. In fact, there's another one coming—but that won't happen until you least expect it.

Just like any good story about an embarrassing moment, this one's going to require a little bit of set-up.

It was 3 AM and time for me to head down to the hotel lobby for my Uber ride to the airport.

"I'm going to need some coffee," I thought. "LOTS of coffee." You must know where this is going. (I don't need to tell you AGAIN, do I?)

My driver was a great conversationalist, but she didn't exactly know how to get to the airport terminal—even with both of our GPS's barking orders left and right.

To make a long story short, I'm two cups of coffee in and stuck in an Uber for forty-five minutes.

When we finally found the Delta terminal, I grabbed my bags and bolted.

But before I could even make it to the doors, I was hit with a sense of panic.

"Oh no! I forgot my phone!"

I was in such a rush that I never unplugged it from her charger.

I turned around just in time to see her pulling away.

I know I must have looked foolish sprinting after her and waving my arms, but I didn't care. My boarding pass was on that phone. Not to mention my family photos, writing ideas, and Clash of Clans village (Hog RIDERS!)

It was no use. Her car was much faster than me (and it had far more gas in the tank.)

Gasping for breath, I looked across the parking lot and saw the airport exit. I sprinted towards that, knowing that she had to go the long way around. As I ran I thought, "This is what I train for."

I sprinted with my bags bouncing off my ankles and watched her distant tail lights get closer and closer to the even-more-distant exit.

Can you guess what happened next?

Anyone?

Yeah. Very good. That's when it happened.

Listen, it was only a little bit. Not enough to run down my leg or anything. Just enough to leave a tell-tale dark spot on my trousers.

Walk. Of. Shame.

Fortunately, I had a sweatshirt that I could pull down far enough to hide my dark secret.

Unfortunately, they make you take off your sweatshirt at security.

They also make you put your hands high over your head while in the body scanner.

There was absolutely no hiding it anymore. Especially because the scanner interpreted the dark spot as a threat to airport security.

What a great time for my first pat-down party with the TSA.

It reminds me of a line from my speech, "Close your eyes. Get ready. I'm going to touch you…" (Incidentally, if you're considering hiring me for an event, that's probably not the first thing you want to show the HR department. They might take it out of context. In fact, just have them skip this entire chapter.)

At some point between the up-close-and-personal inspection and pat down of said area and the rubber-glove-and-cotton-swab test to determine if any chemical weapons or exploding underpants were involved, (Nope. Just an A-bomb to my ego.) I had a realization. I'm the guy who wrote *Magic Words* and *The Four Levels of Influencing People*. I should be able to talk my way out of anything, right?

Thinking quickly, I said to the already uncomfortable agent…

"I peed myself."

Because the first step is always to admit it.

THE FIRST STEP

Admitting that I peed myself was hard. Even if this book only ever sells tens of copies instead of thousands or millions, it was still difficult to put that moment in print. However, admitting to myself that I had a problem with my phone was even more difficult.

After all, this is not an easy thing to pin down. What does it even mean to have a "problem" with my phone? Is it because I use it too much? Well, how much is too much? And who gets to decide that? What if phones aren't as bad as some people say? Besides, isn't everyone else using their phones just as much as I am?

Here's what I realized after I got over the initial shock of losing my phone. I sort of *enjoyed* not having it around all the time.

Without my phone I was incredibly focused, calm, productive, and—perhaps most importantly—PRESENT with the people I love. For a brief moment, I considered going full Amish. I finally understand what Weird Al means by "Amish Paradise." I hate to break it to you, Ezekiel, but his mind is NOT gone. Fool.

For those suffering from "Nomophobia" (the "no mobile phone phobia" in which patients "exhibit excessive phone proximity-seeking behavior") or "FoMo," (fear of missing out) or "FoBo," (fear of being offline) I have good news. I didn't die once. Not one single time. Not only was I still alive, I could actually *feel* it.

Then, after four blissful days of feeding the chickens while Jacob plowed, a package arrived in my mailbox. All at once it was as though we'd never been apart. I fell right back into my old routine and began racking up screen time just like in the old days.

To me, a "phone problem" is when your phone starts taking over areas that you don't really want it to. (More on this in Chapter 5: Are You Addicted to Your Phone?) The thing is, people seem to have a terrible time figuring out what they really want.

Let's go to the polls for a few examples. According to a survey conducted by consumer electronics company, *Retrevo*, forty-nine percent of people are willing to be distracted by their phones during meal time. Twenty-two percent of those polled are willing to (admit to) have a work meeting interrupted by a buzzing device and twenty-four percent won't use the bathroom without their phone in hand. *McCann Worldgroup* played a massive game of "Would you rather…?" with over 7,000 young people. They found that fifty-three percent of kids would rather lose their sense of smell than lose their technology.[1] Another survey of over 1,100 individuals found that forty-three percent of young adults bring their phones into the shower, and that seventeen percent has even checked their phones during sex.[2]

---

1 McCann Worldgroup: Truth About Youth - Conducted in 17 markets, The Truth About Youth is a global study that explores key truths that unite and motivate the Millennial Generation. *https://www.scribd.com/doc/56263899/McCann-Worldgroup-Truth-About-Youth*

2 SureCall Survey - The Attachment Problem: Cellphone Use In America *https://www.surecall.com/docs/20180515-SureCall-Attachment-Survey-Results-v2.pdf*

Device distraction affects many areas of our lives, but none more serious than those times when we're driving a 2,000-pound car. The U.S. Department of Transportation, National Highway Traffic Safety Administration reports that hundreds of fatalities occur every year due to drivers being distracted by cell phones. People are literally dying to check their phones.

There's no doubt about it, our phones have us wrapped around their fingers (or more appropriately, our fingers wrapped around them.) It's time we changed that classic children's song to include the phrase, "The hand bone's connected to the…cell phone." Millions of people are prioritizing their phones over food, sex, relationships, money, work, bodily functions, and even life itself.

You might be shaking your head at how OTHER people interact with their phones. You might feel like you're surrounded by mindless phone zombies. You might even say to yourself, "*I'D* never choose my phone over my most basic needs." You might even be right. But that's not the worst part of the problem. Phones aren't just invading our choices. They're invading those times when your brain is operating on auto-pilot. Those times when you're *not* choosing.

Have you ever driven to work and wondered how you got there? Have you ever put the cereal in the fridge and the milk in the cabinet? Do you consciously have to think about how to move your hand and arm while you're brushing your teeth? Your brain is on auto-pilot like this for about half of your waking time[3]. It's perfectly normal. In fact, it's necessary. The brain's Default Mode Network has evolved to handle routine tasks quickly and more efficiently, saving the heavy lifting of conscious thought for other tasks. It's why you never forget how to ride a bike. It's how

3 A Wandering Mind Is an Unhappy Mind Matthew A. Killingsworth, Daniel T. Gilbert *https://science.sciencemag.org/content/330/6006/932.abstract*

a musician can "feel" the music while playing, and not have to think about it. In fact, thinking about it would likely cause the musician to make a mistake. Concert pianist, Vladimir Horowitz used to say, "The worst thing that can befall a concert pianist is to think about the position of his fingers."

That's the part of the brain that is most vulnerable to racking up extra screen time. Have you ever found yourself swiping through your apps without knowing why you picked up your phone in the first place? Have you ever "felt" a phantom phone in your pocket? (That's when you feel a buzz but your phone isn't even there.) Have you ever looked up from a gaming binge, a Netflix marathon, or a YouTube rabbit hole and then stare at the clock in disbelief? Where did the hours go? I didn't mean to waste so much time! Of course you didn't. We are not really choosing our phone time. It is choosing us. If you were choosing to use your phone so much, then you could simply choose not to use your phone so much. Bad choices are easy to fix. Bad habits are harder.

This is why the digital tide is eroding our happiness, our productivity, our relationships, and our human-ness. And this is why we're letting it happen. I didn't want to admit defeat, but is it possible? Are these little electronic rectangles *winning*?

If they are, then there's really no big mystery why. Just look at the tale of the tape. In that corner, we've got the greatest minds employed by the world's largest companies, with massive budgets, all developing devices and software with one goal in mind: **user engagement**. That's a euphemism for "keeping your eyeballs glued to their screens for as long as possible."

That's why YouTube auto-plays the next video. That's why Facebook uses everything it knows about you to populate your newsfeed with highly scrollable content. That's why Twitter adds a delay before they show you how many notifications you've got (during the delay, your brain anxiously anticipates a reward and actively releases the same feel-good chemicals as when a crack addict takes a hit or a compulsive gambler pulls the arm of a slot machine). That's why the CEO of Netflix says that their "biggest competitor is sleep" and why Candy Crush never ends. None of this is there to serve *you.*

Technology changes quickly. But whether it's social media, virtual reality, the Internet of things, artificial intelligence, wearable (or implantable) tech, or advanced robotics, the company's goal is for you to use their product over and over again without even thinking about it. Compulsively. Obsessively. Relentlessly. And so far, they're undefeated.

In this corner, we've got your brain. Designed and honed by millions of years of evolution to crave the approval and attention of others, to desire significance, to seek reward, escape discomfort, and enjoy novelty. To be fair, it gets into the ring. It sets New Year's Resolutions, reads books, and promises to smoke less, exercise more, and of course, use technology less often. But it's had a rough career. It's got a record of about zero wins and about a thousand losses. I tried to get an exact number of your personal failures, but your mother-in-law was busy. Whatever it is, we all know that when it comes to trying to overcome the pull of technology, the human brain's record is pretty close to unfeated.

Be honest. Who would you bet on?

Even if your phone isn't buzzing, blinking, or chirping, it has likely taught your brain to "self-interrupt." That means that by consistently interrupting you, your phone has conditioned your brain to expect it—to crave it, even. You've been trained like Pavlov's dogs. You check your phone for no reason at all.

Sure, devices are stealing our time. Sure, we're being distracted from important tasks. But that's not what really scares me. What scares me is what technology is in position to do next. Devices are slowly stealing away from us the only thing that matters in life and we're not only letting it happen, we're hurrying the process along.

THE BEST "MEANING OF LIFE" ANSWER OF ALL TIME

Harvard did it. In the 1930's, a team of researchers set out to use modern science to discover the true meaning of life. It was not an easy task. First, they needed hundreds of test subjects to agree to let the researchers pry into their personal business for their entire lifetimes. They managed to get close to three hundred male sophomore students to participate. Because the researchers didn't know what they were looking for, everything had to be measured. Income level, length and number of marriages, work history, physical attributes, demeanor, psychological profiles, genetic makeup, childhood history, life span, and on and on. Everything that could be measured on a man was measured. Yes, even that. ("Size doesn't matter," so sayeth Harvard University.)

Mountains of data were accumulated. When computers came along, those rooms full of information on each subject were analyzed for patterns. Now, after the longest and most comprehensive psychological study in history (over 80 years and $20 million) we have an answer. Harvard cracked the code and gave us the true meaning of life on a silver platter.

Knowing and applying it will make you happier, healthier, live longer, be better at your job, stay married longer, earn gobs more money, and enjoy a host of other benefits.

I'll let George Vaillant, the director of the study from 1972-2003 tell you what it is:

> "The conclusion of the study is that connection is the whole shooting match. The more areas in your life you can make connection, the better. Full stop."

That's it? Human connection? *REALLY?* What about job skills? What about education level? What about a happy childhood? What about natural-born talent? What about exercise and nutrition? What about faith or religious practices? Race? Gender? Life events? Kindness? Accomplishments? Intelligence? Grit? Mindset? Personality type? *Good looks???*

Nope, nope, nope, and nope. They all can help, but on this planet, and in this lifetime, nothing trumps human connection. Some would vehemently argue for their religious beliefs here, but even most major religions contain a strong "love thy neighbor" component and place a significant importance on connecting with others. If you've ever been to a Christian wedding, for example, you have likely heard First Corinthians read by a nervous relative: "And if I give all my possessions to feed the poor, and if I surrender my body to be burned, but do not have love, it profits me nothing."

Is this really a big surprise? Apparently so. One research team from another educational institution conducted a similar study and they were shocked by the results.

"85% of your financial success is due to your personality and ability to communicate, negotiate, and lead. Shockingly, only 15% is due to technical knowledge."

In other words, it's now WHAT you know—but it's also not WHO you know. Rather, it's how well you can *connect* with the people you know and how well you can interact with them. That study was done by the Carnegie Institute of Technology. No wonder why they were so shocked. As an institute of technology, they were probably hoping that technical knowledge would have had a better showing than fifteen percent.

Maybe what's shocking isn't that human connection is important. Maybe what's shocking is just HOW important it is.

Harvard grad and bestselling author, Shawn Achor shows that, "There is a .71 correlation between social connection and happiness. That's nearly *twice as strong* as the correlation between smoking and cancer."

I volunteer at a suicide prevention hotline. Rarely can people be described as "happy" when they call us. Part of my job is to check off the reason the person felt the need to call. Consistently, along with "depression," the "loneliness" and "relationships" columns are often the most full. It seems that when you take away human connection, it affects us in profound ways.

The research goes on and on. People who feel connected to others at home and at work are happier, healthier, more successful, more creative, live longer, earn more, more energetic, more productive, and smarter.

As someone who travels the country speaking to companies on the importance of human connection in a digital age, I can attest. It's not the boxes on the org chart that matter. It's the lines between them. Connection beats talent, hands down. Take the most talented team in the world, but remove human connection and you'll eventually end up with high turnover, low motivation, poor customer service, low sales numbers, a lack of innovative ideas, sloppy execution, an inability to handle change or pivot, and a host of other expensive and frustrating challenges. Exactly how to create a human-connected work culture is beyond the scope of this book. What's important to know is that human connection affects every area of our lives. Even—perhaps especially—the cold, calculating world of businesses and bottom lines.

And what about the *real* bottom line? One of my favorite speaking engagements was for an association of professionals who provide palliative care. These are end of life services such as hospice care and let me tell you, these people deserve a medal every single day. After presenting the closing keynote presentation for half a dozen or so of their state-level events, I got to know a little bit about their world.

There is no one with a better perspective on life on this Earth than someone who is about to leave it. When you sit with someone on their death bed, you learn quickly that accomplishments, acquisitions, accolades, and authority aren't important to them. At the end of our lives, it won't be our collections that matter, but rather our *connections*. We'll spend our final moments thinking about the relationships that we've made or the relationships that we've neglected. They say hindsight is twenty/twenty and those who have that crystal-clear, unclouded perspective are most often focused on human connection.

This makes me wonder, if human connection is going to be what's most important at the end of our lives, then shouldn't it be what's most important now?

Why isn't it?

THE BIGGEST THREAT OF THE TWENTY-FIRST CENTURY

"We know now that in the early years of the twentieth century this world was being watched closely by intelligences greater than man's and yet as mortal as his own. We know now that as human beings busied themselves about their various concerns they were scrutinized and studied, perhaps almost as narrowly as a man with a microscope might scrutinize the transient creatures that swarm and multiply in a drop of water. With infinite complacence people went to and fro over the earth about their little affairs, serene in the assurance of their dominion over this small spinning fragment of solar driftwood which by chance

> or design man has inherited out of the dark mystery of Time and Space. Yet across an immense ethereal gulf, minds that to our minds as ours are to the beasts in the jungle, intellects vast, cool and unsympathetic, regarded this earth with envious eyes and slowly and surely drew their plans against us."

It was the night before Halloween, 1938 when Orson Welles read those words over the radio airwaves to his unsuspecting audience. For the next hour, fake "live" news reports interrupted the musical stylings of Ramón Raquello and described a worldwide alien invasion of cataclysmic proportions. It is said that a mass panic erupted.

And why not? Aliens from Mars releasing poison gas in New York City and killing everyone else with heat rays is a terrifying thought in any decade. Countless movies have been filmed with alien invasion as their main theme. From horror films like *Aliens* and *Signs*, to action flicks like *Independence Day* and *Cloverfield*, to comedies like *Men in Black* and *Coneheads*, to the family-friendly *Gremlins* and *E.T.*, to oddball titles like *Zombies of the Stratosphere* and *Earth Girls are Easy*, to at least a half-dozen adaptations of H.G. Wells' original *War of the Worlds*, it's a fact of human nature. Most people are afraid of aliens.

But not me. In fact, an alien invasion might just be the one thing that can save us from the biggest threat of the twenty-first century. Compared to what's happening now, an alien invasion might feel like a vacation.

When Orson Welles was pranking the population with his War of the Worlds broadcast, Fred Rogers was ten years old. I don't know if he tuned in, but if he did, I doubt he panicked.

"When I was a boy," Fred says, "and I would see scary things in the news, my mother would say to me, 'Look for the helpers. You will always find people who are helping.'"

Calamity brings connection. Shared struggle turns into trust and rapport. Hard times bring people together.

Have you ever noticed how quickly humanity comes together whenever Earth is threatened in the movies? For a real-life example, have you ever noticed how quickly countries come together when threatened by a natural disaster or an opposing army? In 2001, after the attacks on September 11th, "United We Stand" became a rallying cry posted on billboards and bumper stickers. In 2013, after the Boston Marathon bombing, "Boston Strong" appeared on tee-shirts and television commercials.

I'm fascinated how professional sports can seem to echo this. Is it a coincidence that a team called the *Patriots* overcame heavy odds to win the Super Bowl the year of the September 11th attacks? Is it a coincidence that the *Boston* Red Sox—who finished in last place the year before and the year after—won the World Series the year of the marathon bombing? Is it possible that when a community shares a struggle, it brings them together and somehow improves their performance on the playing field? No one knows for sure, but there are a number of interesting occurrences of the teams of affected cities winning the big game.

- 1989—The Loma Prieta earthquake rocks California's Bay Area. The Athletics win the World Series.
- 2001—The US gets hit with the worst domestic terrorist attack in American history. The underdog team named the Patriots wins the Super Bowl.

- 2005—Hurricane Katrina decimates the city of New Orleans and displaced the Saints for more than a year. The Saints won their first home game back at the Superdome in dramatic fashion and went on to make it to the NFC championship game, despite only winning three games the entire previous season.
- 2011—The deadliest tornado in Alabama history tears through Tuscaloosa. The Alabama Crimson Tide win college football's national championship in a decisive blowout.
- 2011—An earthquake and tsunami leave over 18,000 dead and missing in Japan. Japan's women's soccer team wins the FIFA World Cup.
- 2013—Terrorists bomb the finish line at the Boston Marathon. The last place Red Sox win the World Series. In 2014, they fell back into last place.
- 2017—Houston suffers severe flooding after Hurricane Harvey. Astros win the World Series.

This is hardly enough of a sample size to claim statistical significance or to be anything more than a curiosity. But one thing does seem certain, shared struggle brings us together, and we are our best selves when we come together.

Despite the scientific evidence and our own intuition about the importance of human connection, we are still notorious for trying to find ways to push it out of our lives. For as long as there have been humans, wars, bigotry, intolerance, self-centeredness, and of course the root of all evil itself, the love of money, have all tried to pit "us" against "them."

These threats still exist, but there is something new that we've never had to deal with before. This is not the kind of threat that brings us together. In fact, it's quite the opposite. This threat has the best chance of any in history to cause the rapid and methodical extinction of human connection. And it has already begun.

> "I fear the day that technology will surpass our human interaction. The world will have a generation of idiots."

Have *you* noticed a generation of idiots?

That damning quote, most commonly attributed to Albert Einstein, seems prescient. But what does it mean to have a "generation of idiots?" This is not an attack on any specific age demographic. In this case, "generation" refers to a period of time, not a group of people. It's a point in history in which we are all living in, young and old alike. Everyone has been affected; and been affected significantly.

Now let's talk about what it means to be an idiot. The rise of technology has coincided with a drop in attention span, working memory, cognitive ability, and social/emotional intelligence. Whether or not our devices have directly caused these drops isn't known for sure yet, but there is most certainly a correlation and enough circumstantial evidence to make me suspicious.

I'll start with attention span because frankly, I may not have you engaged for much longer. In the year 2000, just before the mobile revolution, Microsoft found that the average adult human attention span was...SQUIRREL!

Okay, I'm back. In 2000, the researchers used EEG to determine that the average attention span was about twelve seconds.

Then, in 2015 the study was repeated, and your attention span is likely one second shorter...*than a GOLDFISH'S*. Critics say that our brain's innate attention *ability* has not changed, just the way we use attention has changed. I say, what's the difference? As the old saying goes, someone who does not read has no advantage over someone who cannot. In either case, attention span *has* been affected. But what about memory?

In the 1950's, Dr. George Miller identified what he called "The Magic Number" as seven (plus or minus two.) This represents the amount of information a typical person can store in his or her working memory at a time. For example, if I were to ask you to remember the number 3407, then you could repeat it in your mind once or twice and have it committed to memory because there are only four digits. However, if I told you to remember 9837465840102766, then by somewhere between the 4's you'd have to grab a pen and start writing it down. Incidentally, this is why phone numbers are seven digits in length. We used to have to remember them. Now, we don't have to remember anything anymore because our phones do it all for us. All I need to do is push a button on my phone and say, "Call my wife" and the phone starts ringing. *I don't even have to remember her name.* Like just about any other skill, if we don't use our memory, we lose it.

Uh-oh. Use it or lose it? We're not using our brains for much of anything anymore! We've outsourced much of our thinking to our devices. In 2010, scientists at McGill University[4] found that "reliance on GPS may reduce hippocampus function as we age." By taking images of the brains of large groups of people, they found that people who used their GPS often had a smaller and less active

4 https://medicalxpress.com/news/2010-11-reliance-gps-hippocampus-function-age.html

hippocampus, the part of the brain most associated with memory. They were also more likely to develop Alzheimer's disease.

Now consider everything else that our devices do for us on a daily basis. We rely on them for much more than just driving directions. We don't have to be smart anymore because our phones are. Any time the title of the song is on the tip of our tongue or any time we wonder how many ants are on this planet, the answer is only a click away. We don't need to figure out how much 17 units at $4.27 each costs because our phones are calculators. Our brains get used to depending on a phone and if there's one around, our brains won't even try. In a 2014 study[5] researchers showed that our cell phone can reduce our performance on complex mental tasks by an average of almost twenty percent—*just by being in sight.* It wouldn't even have to ring. The "mere presence of a cell phone," they said, is enough to make us more stupider.

(By the way, ants not only outnumber us by about 1.6 million to one, but they *outweigh* us. That's fascinating. And it's disgusting. Oh yeah, and the song you were trying to think of was *You Don't Know You're Beautiful*, by One Direction.)

I wonder...what other parts of our brains are shrinking?

I'm going to put a graph below. This graph represents human empathy over a thirty-year period surrounding the rise of smartphone technology and social media. Empathy is the ability to imagine what another person is feeling, and to care. It's important to note that this meta-analysis was conducted by well-respected research psychologist, Sara Konrath. Over 14,000 people were evaluated and all data was self-reported. It has been published in

5 The Mere Presence of a Cell Phone May be Distracting by Bill Thornton , Alyson Faires , Maija Robbins , Eric Rollins *Social Psychology* Nov 2014, Vol. 45, Issue 6, pp. 479-488

scientific journals, well peer-reviewed, and as close to objectively factual as information like this can be. (You can take your own empathy test at www.7DayDigitalDiet.com/tests.) When you're ready, have a look at Figure 1.

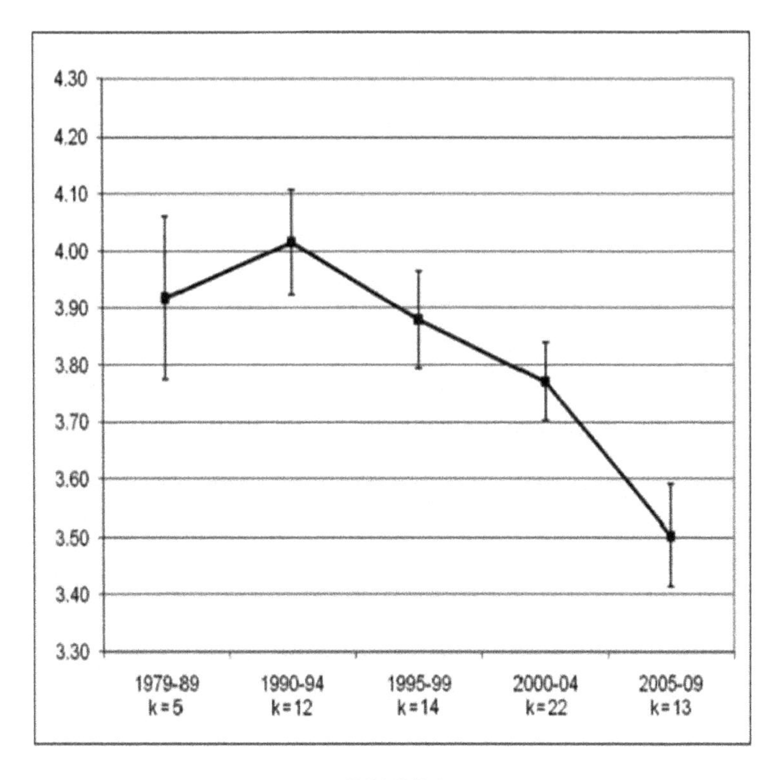

FIGURE 1

Notice that the sharpest decline occurs between 2004 and 2009. This is the same time period when social media sites like Facebook (2004), YouTube (2005), and Twitter (2006) exploded and when the number of text messages sent surpassed the number of phone calls made for the first time in history (2007). That trend has continued to a point where it seems that everyone would rather text than talk. I saw a post on Instagram (2010) that summed it up with a bit of humor.

TIERS OF FRIENDSHIP:

1. We can hang out.
2. We can travel together.
3. I'll take a bullet for you.
4. I will speak to you on the phone.

It's use it or lose it, and our social skills seem to be turning into dust as we push them out in favor of automation and artificial intelligence. Unfortunately, our social skills are not only important in life, they're also pretty important at work. As robots, software, and outsourcing have chipped away at the American workload, human social skill has become more and more in demand (See figure 2).

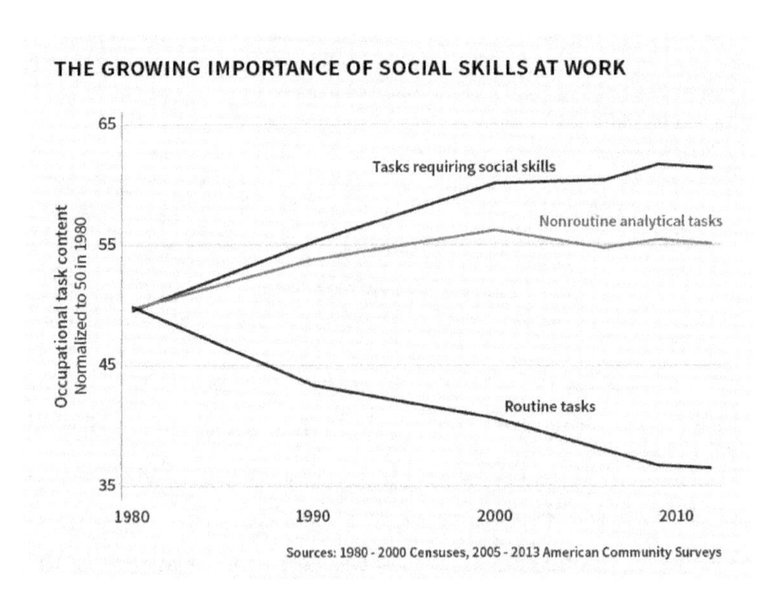

FIGURE 2

Our greatest adaptation is our ability to work together to accomplish incredible things. We simply can't afford to lose it. Especially because since 2009, technology has done just about everything except slow down. Instagram, TikTok, Pinterest, Vine, Snapchat, Tinder, Twitch, and much more have been added to the social sphere and new technologies like live streaming, augmented and virtual reality, voice-controlled devices, the Internet of Things, and artificial intelligence continue to grow. Humans consume more data every year than the previous year, PLUS all other years in history *combined.* Tech isn't going anywhere any time soon. Nor should it have to.

It isn't the rise of tech that worries me. It's the fall of human connection. We aren't just distracted by technology, we are willingly and systematically replacing our moments of interaction with screens, devices, and robotics.

Remember the first time a computer (Deep Blue) beat the world's best chess player (Garry Kasparov) back in 1997? Or how about when IBM's Watson badly beat Jeopardy's best champions in 2011? Well, add another tally to the robot column. With an addition to Google Assistant, dubbed "Duplex," Google aced the never-before-passed Turing Test. It's a piece of technology that pretends to be a human—and gets away with it. The developers' goal was to create something that could make live phone calls for you. The video of Duplex's introduction to the world went viral. Some were amazed, and others were horrified. During the demonstration, the artificial intelligence called a hair salon and booked an appointment for someone named Lisa. It (she?) answered questions and responded to comments in real time. It even interjected the occasional "um" and "uh" in order to better fool the salon employee into believing she was speaking with another human.

What's the problem with that?

It's not the inevitable increase in annoying calls from robot telemarketers, the threat of robots stealing your job, or the possible cyber-crime applications, that bother me most. In my opinion, the worst part of this is the blow suffered to human connection. It's yet another person-to-person interaction that has been removed and replaced with a screen or an app. If we keep doing this, our human-to-human skills will atrophy even more than they already have. Technology continues to bring far people close and close people far. The quantity of connectivity goes up, but the quality of connection comes down.

Duplex is helpful if you're at work all day and can't book your own appointments during normal business hours; but it's harmful if people start using this technology to make ALL their phone calls. What if we get so bad at interacting (or so lazy) that we choose not to even bother? "Okay Google, call Lorraine and tell her she's fired." "Okay Google, call Jim and give him my condolences on the loss of his mother." "Okay Google, call my husband and tell him I want a divorce." What if we start to *choose* technology over the real thing?

What if it's already happening?

Aibo is the name of the robot dog that will replace your living pet. After all, why bother with an animal that sheds, bites, eats, messes on the carpet, and inconveniently dies on you just as you were getting attached to him? *Aibo* can simulate all the benefits of a real puppy, with none of the drawbacks.

Buddy is the robot companion that will replace your friends. This friend will never stab you in the back, gossip about you, or steal your girlfriend. He's always happy to see you and he's got the cutest little face. *Buddy's* IndieGogo campaign raised over $618,000. People want this.

Roxxxy is the realistic robot girlfriend who can hold a conversation and perform all the "acts" that your real girlfriend can, only better. Leave the toilet seat up? No problem. Ask her where she wants to go eat and you'll get a direct answer—without a fight. She has an insatiable libido and never has a headache—unless you enable the "hard-to-get" setting. Do you see why *Roxxxy* flies off the shelves at nearly $10,000 a unit? Do you see why Dr. David Levy (author of *Love and Sex with Robots*) predicts that by the year 2050, human beings will legally be allowed to *marry* robots? He's not alone and many think it will happen sooner. In fact, *Vinclu* is a Japanese company that manufactures Gatebox, an Amazon Echo-like home assistant with a holographic image of an animated woman. By November 2018, they had already distributed over 3,700 "cross-dimension" marriage certificates. The government doesn't recognize them as official marriages yet, but the customers themselves seem to take their relationships very seriously. "I never cheated on her," said Akihiko Kondo, a man who married his Gatebox and spent over two million yen on the ceremony and matching rings. "I've always been in love with Miku-san. I've been thinking about her every day."

Then there are "grief bots." These futuristic robots seem like they walked directly out of an episode of *Black Mirror* or *Electric Dreams*. They are designed to look like your deceased loved one, their personality is re-constructed from their social media profiles and online activity, and recordings of their voice are fed into a software program that can duplicate their voice exactly. The end-result gives you the ability to have a real-time, in-person conversation with something that looks like your dead spouse, sounds like your dead spouse, and acts like your dead spouse. Today, these are being sold as a tool to help surviving loved ones grieve. In the future, these bots will be part of the family dynamic. Why put up with someone's annoying habits when you could just reprogram them?

Has technology gone too far?
If so, can the genie ever be
put back into the bottle?

It's one thing to remove or replace tiny moments of human interaction. The small talk before the meeting, comments about the weather while waiting in line or riding the elevator, and dinnertime conversations have all become opportunities for silent, isolated screen staring. A *Microsoft* research study showed that over 77% of people age 18-24 agreed with the statement, "When nothing is occupying my attention, the first thing I do is reach for my phone." Shared experiences are becoming individual experiences. "A chicken in every pot" got Hoover elected, but "I'm going to build a wall" got Trump elected. But our deepest and most personal relationships are also being replaced. We used to reach out to one another in times of trouble, now we reach for our devices. "Real" is losing its value. And when that happens, what's the value in being human?

What about you?

ARE YOU ADDICTED TO YOUR PHONE?

Let's find out with the following quiz. Read the question and then choose from the responses provided.

Is your phone the first thing you touch every morning and/or the last thing you touch every night?

- Yes
- No
- Yes, but only because it's my alarm.

Throughout the day, do you randomly touch yourself in order to feel the reassuring presence of your phone?

- Yes
- No
- Yes, and I enjoy it.

When you lose your phone, do you lose your mind?

- Yes
- No
- Yes, I can't even poop without it anymore!

Which is worse...getting an amputation or not having a phone for a month?

- Amputation is worse
- No phone is worse
- It depends on which body part.

When your phone's battery is low, do you scout power outlets the way Jason Bourne scouts exits?

- Yes
- No
- Listen, if my phone is dead, then I'll unplug an old lady's life support just to charge it.

Have you ever fallen asleep while holding your phone?

- Yes
- No
- Yes, I actually fall asleep spooning it.

Have you ever ended a phone call because you were driving?

- Yes
- No
- Yes, but only so I could catch up on email.

Okay, that's not the real test. That was just a bit of fun before we dive into a serious topic. Incidentally, you might be surprised at how often people consider getting an amputation if it would mean keeping their phone for the month. Or how many people refuse to even enter a bathroom without a phone in their hands—no matter how bad they have to go. Fortunately, no one is admitting to unplugging life support machines just to make room for their phone charger.

A less amusing, but more legitimate "Smartphone Compulsion Test" was developed by Dr. David Greenfield. He created it to help us determine whether our digital habits are normal and harmless, or problematic. If you'd like, you can take this test right now at: www.7DayDigitalDiet.com/tests.

Greenfield's site states that, "No medical or psychiatric diagnosis can be made solely by a written test." So, it won't tell you directly whether you're addicted or not. But there is a result labeled simply, "Qualifies for a psychiatric evaluation." What does that mean, exactly?

The remainder of this chapter has one goal. To help you decide for yourself how you want to go about labeling your smartphone behavior. I'll present some objective data, debunk some common myths about addiction, and of course I'll recommend that you should always consult with a professional. Addiction is one of those tricky words that not everyone can agree on a definition for. People seem to either fall into the finger-wagging, techno-phobic Luddite camp, longing for the good old days when kids would spend hours playing outside with nothing but a stick. Or they fall into the group that hears the phrase "tech addiction" and dismisses it with a quick "Okay, Boomer" before getting back to consuming tidal waves of data to the exclusion of all else.

The current conversation surrounding tech addiction is either putting too much emphasis on its dangers, or not enough. Specifying the issue for yourself (or discovering that there isn't an issue) is a significant first step. Naming it will help you to tame it.

The word "addiction" was originally used to describe slavery. In Ancient Rome, if you couldn't pay your debts, you'd be sentenced to addiction. After that, the word evolved to mean any bond that is difficult to break. Then in the 1800's (shortly after we learned how to make cocaine,) the term began to refer specifically to substance abuse. Now, two hundred years later, the definition of addiction is changing again.

And what is that definition, exactly? A heroin habit is something we can all point to and agree is an example of addiction. But what about binge eating? There's nothing wrong with food, is there? You're breathing right now. Does that mean you're addicted to oxygen? What about those constant thoughts you're having about your new romantic partner? Does it mean PM Dawn, Cher, Lil Wayne, Candice Glover, U2, Ryan Adams, Beyoncé, and countless others are addicted to their lovers because they sing, "I'd die without you?" If you love art, or baseball, or video games, or music, or sex; then are you addicted? Or does it just mean that you are passionate about something? What makes something an addiction instead of just a habit, passion, or compulsion? And how will understanding this help us to live better?

THE FREQUENCY MYTH

Is something considered an addiction just because you do it a lot? If so, then how much is too much? This is a tricky one because many addiction tests and evaluations—including the one I mentioned earlier[6]—have questions involving how often you consume a substance or engage in an activity. Some think that if you can't go three days without doing something, then you're an addict. But if frequency were the only indicator of addiction, then you'd be addicted to blinking and water. Frequency often correlates with addiction (hence the subtitle of this book) but there are other contributing factors. If you try to combat addiction by only reducing frequency (AKA "cutting back") then you will fail.

THE MINORITY MYTH

There are some who argue that if the majority are indulging in something, then how can it be called an addiction? At that point, it's just human nature and the word "addiction" becomes meaningless. After all, everybody's doing it, right? Adam Alter responds to this idea in his fantastic book, *Irresistible: The Rise of Addictive Technology and the Business of Keeping Us Hooked.* "When, in 1918, a flu pandemic killed seventy-five million people, no one suggested that a flu diagnosis was meaningless. The issue demanded attention precisely because it affected so many people, and the same is true of behavioral addiction." Someone can be an addict AND also be in the majority. Sorry kids, "everyone else is doing it" isn't valid logic if you're trying to convince your parents—or yourself—that something is okay.

6 Dr. David Greenfield's Smartphone Compulsion Test: www.7DayDigitalDiet.com/tests

THE BLAME-THROWER MYTH

"If I kidnap you, tie you down, and shoot you up with heroin for two months, I can create the physical dependence and withdrawal symptoms—but only if you go out and use after I free you will you actually become an addict." That's Maia Szalavitz, author of *Unbroken Brain: A Revolutionary New Way of Understanding Addiction*. This may sound crazy. After all, only five percent of heroin addicts manage to get clean and stay clean. It's one of the most addictive substances on the planet. But having it in your system for two months won't turn you into an addict? What gives?

Unfortunately, there is a small body of animal research that seems to confirm this. One monkey, for example, was locked in a cage and regularly given heroin but displayed no addictive behavior once released from the cage. The physiological effects of the drug alone weren't enough to turn the monkey into an addict. No one knew if the same was true for humans until the 1970s.

In 1971, in a scene straight out of *Breaking Bad*, real-life Asian Walter Whites (master chemists from Hong Kong, hopefully wearing Heisenberg hats) developed a way to make heroin that was 99% pure. Shortly thereafter, the good stuff found its way to US soldiers stationed in nearby Vietnam. It was everywhere. In interviews, eighty-five percent of returning soldiers said they had been offered heroin, many times for free. One dealer would even sneak vials into soldier's pockets and packs hoping they would use it and return for more. Thirty-five percent admitted to trying it and nineteen percent said they had become addicted. Nixon was terrified that the soldiers would bring the problem home with them and the United States would become infested with junkies. He went on national television and declared a war on drugs. His fear turned out to be unwarranted. Upon returning, ninety-five percent of the soldiers who used got off heroin and stayed off. That's an incredible *nineteen times* the typical recovery rate for the drug. The war on drugs didn't even get a chance to start. It didn't have to. Just like with the monkey, drug use alone (even the strongest heroin) wasn't enough to turn the soldiers into addicts. Once they left the cage of Vietnam, the soldiers stopped showing signs of addiction.

The fact is, no one can turn you into an addict. Addiction isn't the result of being exposed to a substance or a behavior. It isn't someone else's fault or responsibility and in the same way, no one can recover for you. You and only you can decide to get better.

THE POPEYE MYTH

For all the good Popeye did to promote eating your leafy green vegetables, his grammar and philosophy about life were left lacking. In just about every episode of his cartoon, you can hear him singing the lyric, "I yam what I yam & dats all what I yam." Really? Then why do you eat spinach? I thought you were what you were. Why try to change your level of physical strength with a performance-enhancing vegetable? Perhaps nurture can have an impact on nature?

You've probably heard the term "addictive personality," or that addiction is a disease. It suggests that some people are just wired to be hooked. It also suggests that addictions are inherently bad and only mentally ill people or people whose brains are somehow broken suffer from them. Though the American Psychological Association still classifies addiction as a disease, the issue has been hotly debated for some time. In 1975 Stanton Peele and Archie Brodsky published *Love and Addiction*, which connected the healthy process of love and attachment to the unhealthy process of addiction. In 1990, a psychiatrist named Isaac Marks said, "Life is a series of addictions and without them we die." In 2005, anthropologist Helen Fisher wrote an article called *Love is Like Cocaine*. Her research involved scanning the brains of addicts and infatuated lovers. There was activity in the same neurochemical pathways in both cases. "Almost everyone on earth feels this passion," she said. Maia Szalavitz, the author we met earlier sums it up beautifully (and also somewhat unsettlingly) in an interview with Adam Alter. "Addiction is a sort of misguided love." In theory, anyone can become addicted to anything at any time. In a way, we're all wired to be hooked because addiction is when very normal (and necessary) brain function goes awry.

If you believe the Popeye Myth, then you may feel like recovery is hopeless. Why bother if addiction is a fixed part of your personality? You "yam what you yam," right? But even if you have the so-called brain of an addict, there is still hope due to neuroplasticity, which is the brain's natural ability to re-wire itself. Don't be fooled by Popeye's outdated philosophy. There is always hope.

THE SUBSTANCE MYTH

In order for something to be considered an addiction, there must be a substance involved, right? Problem gambling, excessive exercise, or binge-watching *Game of Thrones* might be called compulsions or even obsessions, but how can we use the term, "addiction" if there's nothing physical to be addicted to?

Neuroscientist and obsessive behavior expert, Claire Gillan says, "As long as a behavior is rewarding, the brain will treat it the same way it treats a drug. Cocaine has more direct effects on the neurotransmitters in your brain than, for example, gambling, but they work by the same mechanism on the same systems. The difference is in their magnitude and intensity." In other words, it is most certainly possible to be addicted—in every sense of the word—to a behavior that does not involve ingesting, inhaling, or injecting any external substances into the body.

In 2013, the APA updated the Diagnostic and Statistical Manual of Mental Disorders (DSM-5), the principle authority for psychiatric diagnoses, to better reflect modern science's new understanding of addictive behaviors. For the first time, "behavioral addiction" is included as an official diagnosis. In addition, the category, "substance abuse and dependence" was replaced with a more general, "addictions and related disorders."

So far, we've learned that addiction is not identified by how often people do it, how many people do it, how long they do it for, which substances people are using, or whether there is even a substance involved at all. But none of that definitively answers the question posed at the beginning of this chapter. Are you addicted to your phone?

> You are if you use your phone more often than you'd like, and you're doing so in order to fill a perceived psychological need.

I've come across many definitions of addiction, but the modern ones all share this common component. The short-term rewards of the behavior are outweighed by its ultimate negative consequences. For example, your brain quickly learns that the buzzing of your phone often makes you feel popular and accepted by others in the moment. The dopamine hit of social interaction is undeniable. It feels good, so you check your phone again and again hoping for more. Soon, your brain will notice all this extra dopamine and conclude that there was some kind of mistake. It starts to compensate by inhibiting its response to the neurotransmitter. This only makes you seek out more. Eventually, your compulsive screen-staring steals away your time, attention, and *ability* to form deep, meaningful human connections in your life. Addiction is a behavior (even ingesting a substance has a habitual behavior attached) that gives a little to you now but takes a lot from you later.

I couldn't possibly know if you're using your phone more often than you'd like, or if you're doing so in an attempt to fulfill a deeper psychological need. Only working with a qualified professional can properly answer those questions. It is possible that your phone use has become a problem that needs to be addressed. With the proliferation of smartphones and the sophistication level of app design and development, I'd bet that it's even likely. As Adam Alter writes in *Irresistible*…

> "The age of behavioral addiction is still young, but early signs point to a crisis. Addictions are damaging because they crowd out other essential pursuits, from work and play to basic hygiene and social interaction. The good news is that our relationships with behavioral

> addiction aren't fixed. There's much more we can do to restore the balance that existed before the age of smartphones, emails, wearable tech, social networking, and on-demand viewing. The key is to understand why behavioral addictions are so rampant, how they capitalize on human psychology, and how to defeat the addictions that hurt us, and harness the ones that help us."

There's no denying it, as a species we struggle to set boundaries with our technology. More people on planet Earth own a smartphone than a toothbrush. If you've noticed technology pulling your attention away from the priorities and people you value, then it's time to do something about it. Enter the 7-Day Digital Diet.

THE 7-DAY DIGITAL DIET

Some people mistakenly believe that tech is an all-or-nothing deal. They think that the only way to fight overuse is to take a jackhammer to their phone, burn the pieces, and dump the ashes into the center of the nearest ocean. They compare it to how an alcoholic can never let a single drop of liquor cross his lips again for the rest of his life.

Don't worry. You don't need to have an FOAO panic attack (fear of Amishing out.) You can keep your phone, I promise. As long as your phone doesn't keep you. (In America you say, "Hold the phone." In Soviet Russia, phone holds you.)

When you fast, you don't eat ANY food. When you do a detox or a cleanse, you stop eating one or more specific things until they are out of your system. When you go on a diet, you radically change the content and quantity of your food. It typically lasts a finite amount of time at which point you (hopefully) segue into long-term healthy eating habits.

These seven days will be like going on a diet. After that, you'll slip into smarter phoning habits. There's no need to detox.

That's because there's a gray area in all of this. There is a healthy balance. Use isn't always abuse. There is a way to take back what technology has taken from you while at the same time, keeping everything that it has given to you.

You. Are. In. CONTROL.

Never forget that.

I'm simply suggesting that you give your relationship with technology a do-over. Hit the refresh button, if you will. Technology is a great servant, but a terrible master. Maybe we'd all be much better off if our smartphones were put back into the friend zone.

Speaking of friends, now would be a great time to invite someone else to join you if you haven't done so already. Individual friends, family, work teams, religious groups, book clubs, classrooms, civic clubs, sports teams, etc. are all great places to find other people who might be interested in using their phones less and connecting with you more. Don't know what to say? Use the invite tool over at www.7DayDigitalDiet.com/resources. Don't have any friends? Hmm...maybe you need this more than I thought.

This is an important moment in your journey. When doing this challenge with a friend, co-worker, or family member, you'll tap into one of your brain's most powerful motivators. The fear of letting someone else down.

It's similar to how skipping a workout is easy when you planned on doing it alone. However, if your friend is expecting to meet you at the gym, then you're MUCH more likely to show up even if you feel like taking the day off.

NAME	CONTACTED?	FOLLOWED UP?	ARE THEY IN?

FIGURE 3

ACTION STEP: Challenge a friend (or group of friends) to join you in this digital diet. Use the table above to keep track of your invitees.

Just like anything else, some people will be more committed to the digital diet than other people will. If your friend drops out, slacks off, or gives up, then you're back to doing this alone. Not the end of the world, but you'll miss out on all those peer pressure and friendly competition benefits. That's why it's a good idea to have more than two people in your challenge group. In fact, the more, the merrier.

A great place to recruit friends into your challenge group is right on social media. Wait. Hold on a second. Are we actually using technology as a tool to help people use technology less? Wow. That's so *meta*. But if you think about it, isn't that the best place to find people who use their phones too much? Just like tall bridges have signs with suicide hotlines and casinos advertise recovery programs for those struggling with gambling addiction, shouldn't the social media streams contain a way out of their bottomless, time-sucking black holes?

ACTION STEP: Post on social media and invite even more people to join you.

Here are a couple of sample posts you can use:

I'm starting a seven-day "use your phone less" digital diet with @yourfriendsname. Who else wants to join us?

Going to be doing @timdavidmagic's seven-day challenge to improve my relationship to technology. Anyone want to do it with me?

Are you on your phone too much? Yeah, me too. I'm doing a seven-day digital diet. Comment "In!" if you want to join.

Okay, you've got the *who*. Let's talk about the *when*. It's time to figure out your start date. Since you're the one who started all this, you'll have to take the initiative. Grab your calendar right now and pick a day, probably a weekend, when you would have the best chance to go without your phone for twenty-four hours. You're only going to need a one-day "phast" (phone fast), but you will need some time to prepare for it.

Got a date picked? Great, now back up six days and mark that day with "Day one of phone challenge." That's when your smart phoning challenge will begin. For example, did you pick Sunday the twenty-sixth for your one-day phast? Then day one of the challenge will be Monday the twentieth. Ask your challenge group if that day is okay with everyone. If not, change the date. If one person is being difficult, then move on without them. Your group is there to support one another. You can't let anyone else's lack of motivation hold you back.

ACTION STEP: Choose a start date that is agreeable for everyone in your challenge group.

What if the day you picked is three weeks away? That's fine! There are two things you can do right now that will help you gear up for your upcoming *7-Day Digital Diet.*

GEARING UP FOR YOUR 7-DAY DIGITAL DIET

Let's take some time before the 7-day challenge officially begins to get an idea of what your phone habits currently look like. We'll do that by using a tracking app and completing a habit loop discovery exercise. Sounds fun, right? I know. You might be tempted to skip this part, but I highly recommend doing this little bit of leg work up front. It will pay off later, I promise.

INSTALL A TRACKING APP

The first thing you're going to want to do during the challenge is assess exactly how far off you are from your ideal relationship with your phone. What cannot be measured cannot be improved, so let's start measuring using a tracking app.

There are several available. How many will depend on when you're reading this and what make and model phone you have. You're looking for something that can track and record the amount of time you spend on your phone each day. Other features and metrics are fine, but that's the primary one. **There's nothing more important than your time.** Visit www.7DayDigitalDiet.com/resources for recommendations, links, and tutorials. Do it now. This isn't a book you just read. It's a book you do.

You may find that your phone time goes down simply because you know that it's being measured. This is called the Hawthorne Effect and it's perfectly normal. Go with it. It's not the main reason we're doing this, but it's a nice little bonus.

ACTION STEP: Install a tracking app.

Before we dive into the next step, a brief explanation of "The Habit Loop" is required.

THE HABIT LOOP

Every habit has three parts, collectively called a habit loop. A cue (or trigger) that gets it started, the routine itself, and the reward you receive. For example, your **cue** to pick up your phone might be boredom. The **routine** is swiping through a favorite cycle of apps, checking notifications and refreshing feeds. The **reward** you receive is a hit of dopamine any time you see that someone has responded to you, mentioned your name in a kind comment, or liked a photo of you.

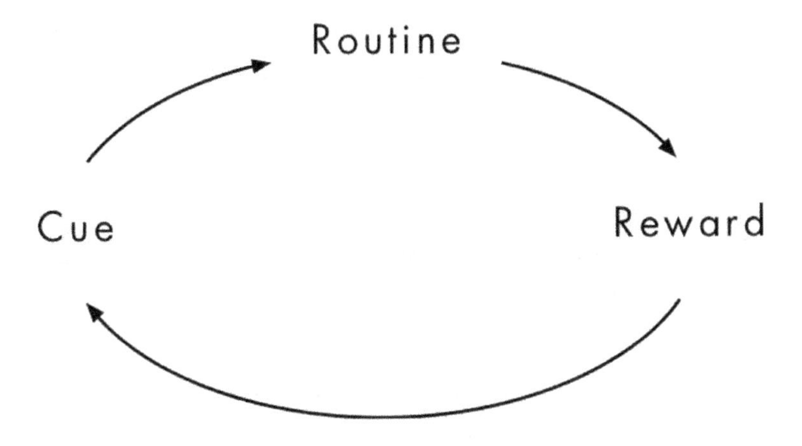

FIGURE 4: THE "HABIT LOOP" AS DESCRIBED BY CHARLES DUHIGG IN THE POWER OF HABIT

Over time, these behaviors may become so ingrained that cravings will develop even when the external cue is not present. You check your phone even when it's not buzzing. That's why it's pictured as a loop. It's a cycle. The more you do it, the more you do it. Back in Chapter 3, the concept of "self-interrupting" was introduced. At first, you would check your phone only when it rang. Eventually, you started checking your phone even if there were no notifications prompting you to do so. The desire for the reward becomes its own cue.

Your brain is wired this way for a reason and it's not always a bad thing. If you're hungry (cue), you eat (routine), and then you feel sated (reward). It's automatic and it's efficient. Much of your day is a cycle of cue, routine, and reward. If you had to consciously think about every cue and constantly make decisions about which routines to engage in, then your brain would be exhausted by noon. Even though our brains only represent about 1.5-3% of our body weight, it consumes about 20% of our energy. Making decisions is metabolically expensive. Your brain requires calories to think just like your muscles require calories to sprint. It's wise for our brains to seek out and execute the patterns of behavior that bring us the greatest rewards with the least effort. Habits are the "light jog" of thinking. But this is also what makes habits potentially dangerous. They become patterns. This is why people will continue in a bad habit, even if they know it's killing them.

GETTING OFF THE HABIT LOOP

Is it true what they say about The Hotel California? That you can check out, but you can never leave? Are we all just prisoners here... of our own device? Absolutely not. Just because it's difficult to get out of the habit loop, doesn't mean it's impossible. Habits can be broken. Addictions can be stopped. Patterns can be interrupted. The habit loop has three parts, but only one of them is your best chance of getting off the downward spiral. Let's look at each of them.

1. **THE CUE.** A German man we'll call "Drünker" had been to rehab over sixty times for alcohol abuse. His cravings were so bad and so constant that he had to have brain surgery. Neurologist, Ulf Mueller implanted an electrical device into his basal ganglia designed to stop the cravings. It worked like ganglia busters. After Drünker recovered from the surgery, images of beers and bars were shown to him. Normally, it would have sent his brain into an tailspin of alcoholic desire, but because of the device, he felt

nothing. Mueller said, "The craving disappeared as soon as we turned the electricity on. Then, we turned it off, and the craving came back immediately." Like Captain Picard, Mueller had gone up against the power of the "cue," and won. It seemed like a miraculous cure for alcohol addiction. The device was left on and Drünker went back to living his life. Things were going fine for a short while until a stressful event brought Drünker right back into the bottle.

What happened? Did the device malfunction? No. It worked perfectly well enough to prevent the ordinary, every day cues from turning into ordinary, every day drinking. But when Drünker experienced that stressful time, his brain immediately sought the reward of relief that booze provided. And when a brain needs a reward, it is likely to engage in a routine that predictably delivers that reward.

The lesson for your own phone habit loop is simple. Don't try to stop the cues. Your phone is always nearby. Technology is everywhere. Everyone around you is using it. It's a part of everyday life and the cues are only going to continue to grow in diversity and in number. Even if you do stop them with brain surgery, it still won't be enough.

"Tim, that's an awfully bleak picture. I thought you said there was hope."

There is. Just not here. Let's go on to where the good news is.

2. **THE ROUTINE.** Bad habits aren't stopped. They are replaced by better habits. A cue will undoubtedly show up. A reward will undoubtedly be sought by your brain. Your

brain is an unstoppable reward-seeking machine. Resistance is futile. Remember, it's part of the healthy programming that has kept our species alive and successful. The good news is that your brain is so focused on getting to the reward that it doesn't care about which routine brings it there.

Drünker started drinking at twelve, was an alcoholic by eighteen, and drank every day of his life. Sixty-plus stints in rehab removed him from the habit loop only by temporarily removing him from his regular life. Surgery eliminated cravings, not the external cues. Neither of those were ever going to work in the way that he needed them to.

That's when he discovered Alcoholics Anonymous. At meetings, and with the help of a therapist, he learned to incorporate new routines into his life other than drinking. The same cues still show up. His brain still demands the same reward. But now he's using different routines to feel better other than alcohol. It finally worked. He hasn't touched a drop since and it's been over twelve years.

This is why we attack habit loops at the routine. This is why we'll be spending the majority of the seven-day digital diet on finding ways to change your current routine while keeping the cues and rewards in place. It's your best hope. A stop sign won't work. You need a detour sign instead. Your brain's reward is still there waiting, but you're going to take a different route to get there. Perhaps you'll discover an even better reward once you're on your new path.

3. **THE REWARD.** Just like you can't eliminate, reduce, or change cues, there's also nothing you can do about your

brain's hard-wired quest for reward. This is why most traditional diets fail. Diets are attempts to deprive your brain of a reward. Even the most dedicated person eventually cheats. Reward-seeking is an unstoppable force. Your best bet is to IDENTIFY the reward that your brain wants, and then find a healthy way to get it.

UNCOVER YOUR CUES AND REWARDS WITH THE STICKY NOTE HABIT LOOP DISCOVERY EXERCISE

If we were to map out your habit loop, the routine would be obvious. It's the *mindless* stuff you do on your phone. It's that app cycle that you hit on a regular basis. You don't even have to think about it. Your thumbs automatically flit to the right spots and before you know it, your device has you in its clutches again. Your tracking software will help to identify exactly which apps are taking most of your time, but for now let's just call the routine, "swipe, stare, and repeat."

Cues and rewards are harder to discover in this case because a mobile device has so many functions and features. There are a lot of reasons we check our phones. Some are important to us, while others are wasting significant time. However, if you had a list of all the times you checked your phone and why, I bet you'd be able to find a few patterns.

There's a very low-tech solution for finding those patterns: Sticky notes. Put a blank sticky note on the back of your phone. Whenever you pick up your phone—and BEFORE you turn it over—write on the sticky note what you're doing, the exact time, and the reason that you checked the phone. You'll need to write really small, abbreviate, or both. Then when you're done, turn the phone face down and write the exact time that you stopped. After a half-hour, your sticky note might look like this:

Lunch - 1:01 - bored - 1:12
Dishes - 1:14 - chk msgs - 1:16
TV - 1:28 - ph buzzed - 1:29

When the sticky note fills up, swap it out for a fresh one. At the end of a day (or a week,) take a look at your sticky notes. You'll likely find times when your phone was acting as a tool to help you do a task. ("GPS," "Unit conversion," "Dan called," etc.) That's what your device is for. We're not trying to reduce phone usage just for the sake of reducing phone usage. We're only interested in minimizing the number of times that our phones waste our time or interfere with our lives in a way that we don't want them to.

Because you'll also see those times when you seemed to be checking your phone for a silly or unproductive reason. Look closely at those. Do any obvious patterns jump out at you? ("Gee, I'm bored a lot.") Can you see common cues? ("Looks like I'm on my phone a lot at work.") What about non-obvious patterns? ("It's interesting how often I check my phone for no apparent reason at all.") What do you think the *real* reward is that you get from swiping through your app cycle? Do some serious soul-searching here. ("Maybe checking to see how many likes I got is just my brain craving the approval of others.")

ACTION STEP: Complete the "Sticky Note Habit Loop Discovery" exercise described above.

CHAPTER CHECKLIST

- Do you have any other people going through the challenge with you?
- Do you have a start date (and a "phast" date) picked out?
- Have you installed a cell phone usage tracking app?
- Have you completed the Sticky Note Habit Loop Discovery exercise?

If so, then congratulations! You're all geared up and ready to begin the seven-day challenge. Let's DO this!

DAY ONE: CHOOSING YOUR TARGET

Are you ready to get to work? I hope so, because I've got a bit of heavy lifting planned for you today. We're doing some of the hard stuff first because I know you've got added motivation right now. This is a new beginning. You're more fired up now than you'll ever be (until you start seeing the results, that is.)

What I'm going to invite you to do next is make or break stuff. The experts agree that if you don't take this action step, then the rest of the challenge is likely to be a complete waste of your time. In other words, it will be worth the heavy lifting. If you haven't been able to reduce your phone use in the past, then this might be your missing link. Think about this…

> This challenge is not about moving away from your phone. It's about moving toward something else—something more important.

For Day One, we're going to identify exactly what that something else is going to be. As an example, one December, every time I caught myself mindlessly picking up my phone, I would force myself to pick up a book and read one full page (or more) before I allowed myself to check my phone. By the end of the month, I had read eleven books!

This is an EXTREMELY important psychological tactic. If you did the sticky note exercise from the previous chapter, then you would have seen that mindlessly checking your phone gives your brain very specific psychological rewards. Your brain isn't going to give them up easily. So, ask yourself this question...

Can you give your brain that same reward in a healthier or more efficient way? Or could you give yourself a better reward altogether?

For example, the reward that my mindless swiping brought me was relief from boredom. But the feeling of accomplishment, not to mention all that I learned, from reading eleven books far outweighed simply passing the time. So that's why I set a target of reading at least one page of a book *before* mindlessly checking my phone.

I can't stress this enough, "use my phone less" is NOT a target. It's a result. When Tiger Woods lines up for a shot he doesn't say to himself, "Don't hit it in the bunker." Instead, he focuses on the green that he's aiming for. When Pedro Martinez was in mid wind-up, he wasn't thinking, "Don't hit this guy." Instead, he was focused exclusively on hitting the catcher's mitt for a strike that paints the outside black. Sports and science have shown us that it is far better to identify what you want instead of what you don't want.

"Never take a shot without a target."
– Earl Woods, father of Tiger Woods.

"Begin with the end in mind." – Stephen Covey, author of the perennial #1 bestseller, 7 Habits of Highly Effective People.

"Start with why." – Simon Sinek, author of Start With Why: How Great Leaders Inspire Everyone to Take Action and giver of the most popular TEDx talk of all time.

For some people, coming up with something to accomplish is a piece of cake. Others have already failed the challenge. Don't worry, I'll walk you through the entire process. By the end of the day, you'll not only have a target you can work towards—one that will give your brain the rewards it craves—but also a written version that will give you the best chance of reaching it.

ACTION STEP: Grab a piece of paper and complete Brainstorm #1: The WHAT.

BRAINSTORM #1: THE WHAT

Fill in the blanks below with the first thing that comes to your mind. Don't edit your thoughts at this point, just allow your mind to dream. It's okay to skip questions, repeat your answers, or copy off your neighbor.

I've always wanted to ___________________________________

____

A book I've been wanting to read/finish reading is ____________

____

A physical activity I enjoy is ____________________________

____

A skill I would like to develop is __________________________

____

A language I'd like to be able to speak fluently is ___________

____

I really miss talking to ______________________________

____

All my life, I've been afraid to ________________________

____

If I ever wrote a book, it would be about ________________

____

A musical instrument I'd like to play more is _____________

____

It's been a long time since I __________________________

____

I'd love to make/build/paint/sculpt a ___________________

____

My creative outlet is _________________________________

____

For fun, I enjoy ____________________________________

____

A topic I'd like to learn more about is __________________

____

I would enjoy volunteering my time for _________________

____

If only I had more time for ____________________________

____

My boss/spouse/friend wishes I would __________________

____ more

My phone gives me this reward_________________________

I could get that same reward better/faster/smarter/healthier by___

____

YOUR ANSWERS MAY INCLUDE THINGS LIKE:

- Working out
- Spending time in nature
- Playing chess
- Learning French
- Feeling gratitude
- Playing piano
- Spending time with my children
- Studying the bible
- Gardening
- Skiing
- Donating blood
- Meditating
- Rock climbing
- Cooking
- Walking/Running/Biking
- Calling mom

I know it is tempting to skip a step like this and keep reading, but I promise, you'll regret it if you do. The single biggest reason people fail when they try to cut back on their phone use is because they don't replace the unwanted activity with a different, target activity. If you did skip Brainstorm #1, then stop reading and go back and do it now. When you're done, it will be time to write down your target in such a way that will give you a significant head start.

PUTTING IT INTO WORDS

I've spent quite a few years studying human motivation and behavior change. One of science's most amazing findings is that tiny differences in the way you *think* about your target can make a massive difference in your likelihood of reaching it. I've created an acronym using the word "PURPOSE" to help you frame your target in a way that your brain can get excited about.

Positive: Tell yourself what you're doing, not what you're not doing. For example, you won't be writing something like, "I don't want to be a lazy, fat phone zombie anymore." You see, that is slightly negative. Go get a hug from someone right now. It is scientifically proven that the brain works much better when things are worded positively[7]. So, instead of saying, "I don't want to be a lazy, fat phone zombie anymore," you would say something to the effect of, "I read for thirty minutes a day."

Unlimited: You will get from yourself whatever you expect from yourself. The only reason I was able to read eleven books that December was because I followed the "unlimited" rule when I set my target. Had I left it at "Every time I pick up my phone, I will read one page of a book instead," then I would have stopped after one page. By adding the words "or more", "or better", or "or faster", to your target, you'll turn off your brain's internal alarm that would otherwise tell you to stop once you've reached it.

Realistic: Think about your likelihood of success here. Is this something that will be doable? Easy, even? Are you an optimist or

7 Planning What Not to Eat: Ironic Effects of Implementation Intentions Negating Unhealthy Habits: http://journals.sagepub.com/doi/abs/10.1177/0146167210390523

a pessimist? A study by psychologist, Gabriele Oettingen showed that obese women who thought their upcoming weight loss program would be easy lost twenty-four pounds LESS than those who thought their weight-loss program would be a challenge. Does this mean that pessimism is the way to go? Not so fast. The purely pessimistic women stayed twenty-six pounds HEAVIER than the optimists.

The key is to be a REALISTIC optimist. Believe that the process will be difficult, but that you will persevere. If you aren't realistic about the challenges that are most certainly coming, then you will be blindsided by them.

If you can't seem to shake your pessimism or your optimism, then it might be time to adjust your target. Choose one that will stretch you, but not break you. In a situation like this, when you're trying to replace an unwanted habit with something better, it's best if your target errs on the side of easy. You don't want to tell yourself that you're going to spend more time in nature if the nearest tree is a forty-five-minute drive from your house. It's simply not realistic to expect that you're going to do that EVERY time you pick up your phone.

Present-Tense: Instead of writing "I am going to," it's much smarter to write, "I speak conversational French." When your target is written like this, you're sort of tricking your brain into believing that you have already achieved it. Newton's first law teaches us that it's much easier to continue doing something than it is to start doing something. I find that this has a way of helping me to change my self-identity. When I think of myself as an avid reader, I'm more likely to act in a way that supports that belief. It's a self-fulfilling prophesy, but there's nothing mystical about it. There's a solid body of neuroscience to back this up.

Orchestrated: Does your new target fit in nicely with other targets you've set in your life? Will working toward that big promotion take time away from your goal of spending more time with your kids? As the old saying goes, when you chase two rabbits, both of them get away. Targets can compete for your mental resources as well as physical. Should you really try this seven-day phone challenge while you're also quitting smoking and starting a new diet? The science (and common sense) says no. Willpower is like an emotion that comes and goes. There are conditions that help bring it about, and conditions that push it away. When you're overwhelmed and stressed, willpower retreats. Like a conductor, your role is to ensure that your new target will add to the symphony of your life and not ruin it or distract from it. You can do anything, but you can't do everything. Set your priorities and tackle your targets in a manner that gives you the best chance of success.

Here's a bit of good news from the world of scientific research: because willpower is like an emotion, it doesn't run out when you use it. Love grows the more you use it. Gratitude gets richer the more you practice it. The same is true for negative emotions like anger or hate. When your willpower is strengthened in one area of your life, it is strengthened in all other areas as well. By focusing on one target at a time, you may notice that your next target also gets a little closer as a result.

Specific: I read a story once where this guy found a magic lamp and when he rubbed it a genie popped out. Only this genie wasn't the nice, Robin Williams genie from Disney's original *Aladdin*. This genie was very passive-aggressive.

The guy wished for more money and the genie gave him a penny. "Well, you asked for more money, you didn't say how much!" Then he wished for a beautiful mansion and he laid out all the specifics. The genie gave him everything that he asked for. The mansion was beautiful and it perfectly matched the guy's description. The only problem was that it was smack in the middle of Antarctica. For his third wish, he took his time describing every imaginable detail for the perfect woman. "I wish that someone like this would fall in love with me!" Sure enough, the perfect woman came along. Only she was only a baby now. Over the years, she grew up to fulfill each of the criteria he had given to the genie. Finally, she professed her love for him. It was the day before he died.

Your subconscious mind is like the genie in the story. Only it's not mean on purpose. It's just very literal and will rise or fall to the precise level of expectation that you set for it. This is why a specific implementation intention is so important. With this phone challenge, you'll be doing two things, minimizing one behavior (mindless scrolling) and maximizing another behavior (your new target.) Psychologists have found that replacement intentions like this are best phrased as if/then statements.

Here are some examples that incorporate the entire PURPOSE acronym so far…

If I have the urge to check my phone, then I'm walking into my kitchen, picking up my new book, and reading one or more pages.

If I hear a text notification, then I'm taking five deep breaths or more and intentionally deciding whether or not I can check my phone guilt-free.

If I open my video game app, then I'm immediately dropping and doing twenty or more push-ups before playing.

If I check email or social media outside of my scheduled times, then I'm briskly walking around the perimeter of my property for one full lap or more.

When you're as specific as possible about the activity, the quantity, and the location, then you paint a picture for the little genie that lives inside your mind. It's always easier to hit a target that you can clearly see.

End Date: The final step is to make sure that you give yourself a deadline. An end date will keep you focused. If you don't give your goal a deadline, it's just a wish that will forever live in the land of "someday." Besides, it's much easier to eat an elephant one bite at a time than in one big gulp. Even *Alcoholics Anonymous*, perhaps the most successful behavior change organization in the world, takes a life-long target (never drink again) and creates a series of specific end dates with their "one day at a time" mantra. Your first end date will be the end of the seven-day challenge.

ACTION STEP: Grab one more sticky note and write down your complete if/then statement with PURPOSE. Then, take a picture of it and set that picture as your new lock screen.

Now you're going to be reminded of your target at the precise moment that you're being tempted by your phone. It's the detour sign that takes you off the habit loop. If your tracking app keeps tabs on how many times you unlock your phone, then take a look at the data you've collected so far. Whatever your average unlocks number is (and I know I was shocked by how high the number was) that's how many times you'll be reminded every single day to replace your unwanted phone routine with those behaviors that will help you reach your target.

Even if that reminder doesn't change your course, it will still act like a speed bump, slowing you down and forcing you to take note of where you're going. Of course, you'll still have the freedom to unlock your phone and use it however you see fit. It's perfectly okay to mindlessly "zone out" on your phone every once in a while. As long as you're making that decision consciously instead of out of habit, then there's nothing wrong with using your phone however you want to use it. It should be about what you want, not about what the habit loop wants.

CHAPTER CHECKLIST

- Have you completed Brainstorm #1?
- Do you have a *written* target using the PURPOSE model?
- Have you changed your phone's lock screen?
- Have you logged today's unlocks and/or screen time?

DAY ONE: DO THIS FOR EXTRA CREDIT...

The right words, in the right place, at the right time. It makes so much logical sense. The only problem is, logic is never enough. We're going to need to appeal to your emotional self as well. To do that, we need a new photo for your phone's wallpaper.

The wallpaper is different from your lock screen. It's the background image behind all of your little square app icons. It's the largest image, but you rarely see it. Let's finally put that space to good use.

Find a visual reminder of your target. You might take a photo of the book you want to finish reading. It might be a photo of the garden that you want to nurture more. It could be of the children you want to spend more time with. Grab something off your vision board. Grab something off the internet. It doesn't have to make sense to anyone else, but the more emotionally charged the image is for you, the better. Brainstorm #2 is designed to stir up some of those emotions.

ACTION STEP: Complete Brainstorm #2.

Even if you're only doing this challenge because someone else asked you to, now is the time to make it your own. Brainstorm #2 will help you to come up with a list of powerful reasons that are all yours. I don't want to hear why "people in general" *should* complete this challenge. I don't want to hear why you *have to* complete this challenge. This is all about what YOU *want*. When you're done, I bet one (or more) of those powerful reasons will be able to be represented by an image. THAT'S the kind of image we're looking for.

BRAINSTORM #2: THE WHY

With this exercise you'll get four related writing prompts. The goal is to formulate a list of reasons why engaging in your target behavior will be more rewarding than swiping and staring at a screen.

WHEN I REACH MY TARGET (GOOD)

This is everything that I will gain when I reach my target. *(Describe all the positive feelings you will experience, and all the positive things that will happen. Get specific. What will people say to you? How will you feel? What will happen? What will you see? Write it all out below.)*

WHEN I REACH MY TARGET (BAD)

This is everything that I will lose when I reach my target. *(There is always something to sacrifice in pursuit of a new target. When trying to reach financial freedom, for example, you'll probably give up the ability to spend frivolously whenever you want. Bummer. But there are also negatives that you might lose such as the embarrassment of always having to say, "I can't afford it." Write it all down.)*

IF I FAIL TO REACH THIS TARGET (GOOD)

This is everything that I will gain if I DON'T reach my target. *(There is likely some kind of reward keeping your brain in its patterned behavior. It's best to know about it so that you can make the conscious decision that everything written below is simply not worth more than what you will gain by achieving it.)*

IF I FAIL TO REACH THIS TARGET (BAD)

This is everything that I will lose if I DON'T reach my target. *(Pain is a powerful motivator. Tap into the pain using your imagination so that you won't have to experience it in real life.)*

What you've just done is shown your brain a compelling case that the reward for engaging in your target behavior is greater than the reward for "swiping and staring" at a phone. Remember, you WILL experience cues that WILL trigger routines that WILL generate rewards. The habit loop marches on. Cues for technology are everywhere and the short-term reward of feeling socially connected and affirmed is enormous. Don't try to convince your brain that a feeling of accomplishment for resisting phubbing your spouse is a good enough reward. That's like trying to convince a six-year-old that giving is better than receiving. It's a good lesson and it might sound good on paper, but in the moment, the kid just wants his presents. That's why his behavior will naturally reflect that unless he's been taught otherwise. Brainstorm #2 *magnifies* the net rewards of skipping the mindless phoning in favor of your target routine. But that doesn't mean you'll do it. The six-year-old won't get it after you tell him once either. Repetition is important if this is going to sink in and create true, lasting behavior change.

ACTION STEP: Convert your most powerful reason into an image and set that image as your phone's background wallpaper.

However, you've likely brainstormed more than one emotional reason to reach your target. Let's not let those go to waste. Choose a few of the more powerful ones, write them down on an index card, and attach the card to a place where you look every day. Maybe it will go on your bathroom mirror, your computer screen, your wallet, or your car's dashboard. Like a loving parent would, you want to gently remind your brain of what is truly important to you—over and over again. Be relentless with your repetition. This is all about getting yourself excited about something that really matters to you on a deep, emotional level.

ACTION STEP: Surround yourself with reminders of your most powerful emotional reasons to reach your target.

What if you mess up? What if nothing changes? What if things get *worse*? That's okay. Don't beat yourself up. **Slipping up is fine but giving up is not.** Stay the course. We're just laying a foundation for now. We've still got six more days as well as an entire chapter called, *What if it Didn't Work?* I've got LOTS more tricks up my sleeve and I promise we'll have fun along the way.

CAUTION: YOUR BRAIN IS GLITCHY

Have you ever driven away with the coffee still on the roof of your car? Have you ever gotten cash back at the self-checkout, but accidentally walked away with the twenty still sitting in the dispenser as a nice surprise for the next person in line? Psychologists call this common brain glitch "post-completion error" and you're in danger of having one right now.

Writing down a target is a step towards an achievement, not an achievement itself. You've simply marked down your starting point, your ending point, and you've had a look at the terrain in between. You've done good work, but don't let your brain accept this as a full accomplishment. If you do, then your brain might think that it's time for a rest when in reality, you're just getting started.

Another possible pitfall is telling people about your target. Saying, "Did you know that I'm writing a novel?" feels good, especially when the other person responds enthusiastically, but it tricks your brain into a post-completion error. You'll have to forcibly remind yourself that all you've done is made a decision to act.

Zig Ziglar would have advised you to, "Tell people your give up goals, but not your go up goals." So, do tell people that you're doing a seven-day smart phoning challenge and they'll help hold you accountable to it, but don't tell them that you're planning on starting a new business. Not only will you be more likely to experience a post-completion error, but they also may throw some toxic negativity at you about the likelihood of your imminent failure.

CHAPTER CHECKLIST

- Complete Brainstorm #2.
- Change your phone's wallpaper.
- Strategically place reminder notes throughout your daily world.
- Avoid post-completion errors.
- Congratulate yourself on doing an amazing job so far!

DAY TWO: THE FAULT IN THEIR DEFAULTS

The first order of business today is to give yourself a treat. Yesterday was tough! Besides, all that talk about rewards... maybe it's time to get one. Remember, if you're going to train your brain in a way similar to training a child or a pet, then chocolate ice cream can be a powerful tool. If you don't like ice cream, pick something else that makes you feel good and indulge a little bit. Self-bribery isn't a technique that is practical for the long-term, but while you're learning a new habit, every little bit of motivation helps!

ACTION STEP: Reward yourself for a job well done so far! Then promise yourself ANOTHER reward when you complete today's action list.

A large percentage of your phone's features go unused. I mean, it's crazy. We spend all kinds of money to have the latest and greatest gadget without truly understanding what makes it so great. Even if you consider yourself tech savvy, someone more tech savvy than you could probably sit down and show you twenty features that you didn't even know existed.

Don't worry, *I'm not that guy.*

I am psych savvy though, and I know that the default settings on your phone weren't put there with your best interests in mind. At best, the developers choose them randomly or arbitrarily. At worst, they are purposefully put in place to get you to watch more, swipe more, tap more, and buy more. Let's face it, your well-being is pretty low on their priority list. Some good features are already on your device, they just don't set them up for you or tell you about them.

It looks like we're going to have to do it ourselves.

The first default setting you can kill right now is excess notifications. I consider anything that does not come directly from another human to be excessive. The notification from a video game telling you that your friend just beat your high score? It's gotta go. The one from YouTube saying that Tim David just posted a new video? Thanks for being a subscriber but turn off that pesky notification. The one that tells you someone just liked your Facebook comment? I know the affirmation feels good, but let it go. It's emotional junk food. The one warning you that a flash flood is imminent in your area? Okay, that one can stay. So can a buzz letting you know that Jim just replied to your direct message asking about dinner plans.

ACTION STEP: Turn off ALL notifications except those that come from selected humans.

A common hang-up with this step is email. What if someone from work tries to get in touch with you about something important? You can't just disappear off the digital map. More likely however, is you'll get an email ding, check your phone, and find that someone claiming to be your long-lost uncle from Namibia has $25,000,000 that he needs your help spending. Was that email really worth your time? No. I'm telling you right now. Your uncle is not M. Ndemufayo, the last king of Kwanyama.

That's why in this action step, you'll be only allowing "selected" humans to make your phone light up. Most email applications and mobile devices allow you to customize who gets onto your notifications guest list, and who has to wait outside the velvet rope. Obviously, you'll still receive all your emails and they'll be there waiting for you when you check. But they'll no longer have an all-access, backstage pass into your pocket.

Imagine what it would be like if you only checked your email three times a day, at scheduled intervals. Imagine how productive and present you could be! Everyone knows that time is our most valuable commodity because it can never be replaced. It's not just the quantity of your time that matters though. It's the quality. It is worth protecting your focused time spent "in the zone." The value that focus adds to your work life and personal life is immeasurable.

You can also take advantage of your phone's built-in "Do not Disturb" settings. This allows you to automatically switch back and forth between being more and less reachable via notifications. For example, maybe you want every notification during work hours, but during the evenings and weekends, you want fewer distractions so that you can focus more on your personal relationships.

You may want fewer distractions regardless.

The more distracted you are by notifications, the more your brain will learn to be distracted easily. You'll end up like Pavlov's dogs, running and drooling every time you hear a bell. And speaking of classical conditioning, after completing this action step, you may find that your brain will continue to "self-interrupt" during those times when you're trying to remain focused. Your mind will easily and quickly wander with or without any external distractions. It's like a phantom limb that still aches even though it has been amputated. In the middle of reading a book, you'll feel an unexplained pull to switch to something else. "Isn't there something I could be checking right now? Email? Sales numbers? Social media? Last night's box scores?" You might even physically *feel* your phone vibrate in your pocket even though it didn't. This just means that distraction has been the norm for long enough to become a conditioned habit.

Turning off notifications and customizing other settings isn't a cure for the distracted brain, but it is an important first step.

CHAPTER CHECKLIST

- Have you rewarded yourself for yesterday?
- Have you turned off ALL notifications that don't come from selected humans?
- Have you put limits on the access that people have to you via email using your email provider's settings, "out of office" replies, and/or your phone's "Do Not Disturb" settings?
- Do you have a plan for how often you will allow yourself to check email?
- Have you patted yourself on the back for completing Day Two?

DAY THREE: CHAAAAAARGE!!!

Your phone is ruining your sleep life.

If there's anything that requires a huge amount of focus, it's sleep. Your brain needs six to nine hours of uninterrupted sleep every night. Most of us think of sleep as a completely unconscious activity, but there are several phases of the sleep cycle including the precious minutes right before you fall asleep and right after you wake up.

Instead of using that "wind down" time for restoration, contemplation, and rejuvenation, many people are staring at their phones straight up until they lose consciousness. The next morning, their phone is the first thing they touch, and the cycle continues. Phoning might seem like a wind-down kind of activity, but the brain doesn't think so. Phones pump stimulating music, video, and social content straight into your eyeballs and earballs. They give you the powerful dopamine hit of "slot machine swiping" and refreshing. Your brain drinks in the constant newness and novelty of the Internet and swims in a cocktail of chemicals as a result. It's like a quiet mini techno rave. Even the blue light emitted by the screen confuses your natural circadian rhythms.

ACTION STEP: Start charging your phone overnight in a room different from where you sleep.

Yes, this means you'll probably have to travel back to 1999 and buy an alarm clock. Don't worry. They're cheap now. Well worth what you'll be earning back in sleep.

Have fun with this. Set up a "charging station" and enjoy the fondness that a little distance between you and your phone can make. Use retail therapy and buy yourself a fancy new charger. See if you can get one in lipstick red. It will be a visual reminder and a cue to begin your new routine. You could even get a small bed for your phone and "tuck it in" every night. A company based in the Netherlands[8] will make one for you. They might be on to something. In addition to the novelty and cuteness factor, the routine of tucking your phone in at night (and singing it a lullaby?) can become a habit itself and therefore you'll be more likely to stick to the plan. Put your pajamas on, brush your teeth, and tuck in your phone. Hey, phones need their rest too.

8 http://www.bug-bed.com

CHAPTER CHECKLIST

- Do you have an alarm clock?
- Have you set up a charging station for your phone in a room different from where you sleep?
- Have you logged today's unlocks and/or screen time in your companion journal?
- Did you have fun with this?

DAY FOUR: DRAG AND DROP

When I was a kid, I had a messy room. I wasn't a hoarder or anything, but it took me a few years to discover that my carpet was blue. Sloppy surroundings don't exactly have the best effect on your mental state. If I had homework to do, I practically needed an excavator to get to my pencil box and TI-82 scientific calculator. While digging for that, I'd come across a Lego piece that I'd been looking for so that I could finish building a bomb shelter for my Star Wars action figures. Not terribly productive. If my room was a bit more organized, then maybe it would have helped to eliminate some of those distractions.

In that way, your phone is no different than a bedroom. App icons are shiny, colorful little squares that are competing for your attention. Some even have notification bubbles popping out of their corners like little hands being raised. Grab your phone right now and have a look at your display. How many apps do you see? How many *pages* of apps do you see? You can almost hear the little things screaming for your attention. You open your phone for one thing, but you end up doing something else entirely.

The goal is to be able to get into your phone when you need to, and then get out before you get sucked into the black hole. Get in. Get out. Done.

ACTION STEP: Organize your phone's display according to the following recommendations.

FIRST PAGE: Some apps are useful tools, not distractions. These are apps that serve a specific purpose and yet, there is no temptation to continue using it after it has served that purpose. For example, a GPS helps you get to where you're going. Once you arrive, you turn it off. You very rarely see people addicted to their GPS units. That's just not a screen you stare at unless you're trying to get somewhere. Maps and driving directions apps are "get in, get out" tools and therefore they are allowed on your home page.

Other examples of tools that you'll allow on your home page are your camera, weather apps, smart home apps (unless you find yourself constantly watching your empty living room via the security camera), banking apps, calendar, notepad, etc. If you can't fit everything on your home page, then by all means, use folders. Organizing apps in folders is strangely satisfying.

SECOND PAGE: This is the page for apps that are both useful AND distracting. The app may serve a practical (or pure entertainment) purpose, but once you're in, it's hard to get out. That's why I call these "mafia apps." An example would be any kind of messaging app. They're helpful for keeping in touch with loved ones, but the chatting might also get out of hand. Sometimes, we just use these to shoot off a quick "Hey" to fifteen people so we can get a wave of social interactions, even if they are phony and fleeting.

Other examples of mafia apps are video games, email apps, shopping apps, social media apps, comedy apps, web browsers, dating apps, news apps, etc. Your decision is simple. Does the app add to the quality of your life? Or does it just feast on your attention? If the positives outweigh the negatives, then stick it on your second page (but hide it inside a folder…we don't want these ruffians running free.) If not, then delete it (relax, you can always reinstall it later) or move it to the third page. If you're unsure, then go to Settings > Battery to see which apps you use the most. That might give you a hint as to which apps are the biggest attention suckers.

THIRD PAGE: The third page is sort of a holding area for the apps you're not quite ready to delete yet. There are a few categories of apps that fit the bill and I'll go through each of them now. Some apps can't be deleted. That's okay. We won't let them win. We'll demote them to the third page and tuck them away in a folder titled something like, "Tyrants," or "Damn the Man." It's up to you, really. The third page will also contain what I call "potentially useful clutter." For example, I've got a ruler app on my third page. (The measuring stick kind, not the um…tyrant kind.) It's *potentially* useful to have a measuring tape in my pocket at all times, and convenient not to have to reinstall an app every time I want to measure something. That's a keeper for page three, just in case. (Now do you see why I used the word "clutter"?) Next, anything I've paid for, but don't often use goes on page three. *Stellarium* is an example. Anytime I'm curious about a bright dot in the night sky, I point *Stellarium* at it to find out what it is. Not worthy of page one or two, but I paid for it, so it isn't worthy of the dustbin either. The last category for page three is apps that you would only use in an emergency. *Find my iPhone* is an example of an app you'd only use in an emergency (or to spy on your spouse).

NO PAGE: It's time to start deleting some apps. This is the "drop" portion of "drag and drop." Anything that takes more than it gives has got to go. That probably means some social media apps, some dating apps, that app you haven't used in four years, the stupid game that you play for three hours a day, and the trendy technology that never took off (I'm looking at you QR reader.) Remember, if you're feeling uneasy about hitting the little "x" and watching the app fade away, it's not gone forever. You can always reinstall it. Also, you can log in to Facebook or Twitter on your computer or phone's Internet browser. You don't have to give up social media, just maybe the app on your phone.

RECOMMENDED ACTION STEP: Sign up for a password manager before you delete any apps.

A password manager stores all your passwords and keeps them secure so that only you can access them using one master password. The advantages are numerous, including only having to remember one password. Most cyber-security experts say that password managers are a good thing too.

THE MENU BAR AND CONTROL CENTER: The menu bar is the row of apps that runs across the bottom of your screen. The control center is what appears when you swipe up. These areas can both most certainly be customized and should be reserved for only the best of the best. That is, the tools you use most often.

Okay, you've tidied up. How do you feel? Hopefully you feel a sense of accomplishment along with a sense of frustration because you can't find anything anymore. That's a good thing. Try to get in the habit of opening apps only by using your search bar. You're less likely to be pulled in to other apps that you weren't intending on using in the first place. It's all about intentional phone use, not the accidental screen stare.

A nice side-effect of not knowing where your apps are, is you get an added speed bump. Instead of quickly and automatically flitting your thumbs across the screen in a choreographed tap-dance, your pattern is interrupted and you're forced to think. That extra moment may be enough to get you to get out of the habit loop. You may want to consider tidying up once a month. If you've got nothing new to drop, then just drag your apps around to new locations. Hide them in folders with strange, unhelpful names. I actually enjoy doing this. It's like playing hide and seek with myself.

CHAPTER CHECKLIST

- Did you set up a password manager?
- Have you organized your icons with intentional use in mind instead of speed, convenience, or color?
- Have you deleted at least two apps? (C'mon, there's no way you need to keep EVERYTHING...)
- Have you started opening apps by using the search bar instead of tapping the icons?
- Have you given yourself a high-five for being awesome?

DAY FIVE: CLAIM YOUR NO-PHONE ZONES

It's time to draw a line in the sand. Several, in fact. There are some areas of your life where your phone is off-limits. There are some moments in your life when your phone is a no-no. No exceptions.

Before you get mad at me for being a dictator, you should know that you'll be making all the decisions and drawing all the lines. Remember, you are in control every step of the way. Every healthy relationship has boundaries and it's time to set a few.

ACTION STEP: Create a list of possible "no-phone-zones."

Driving. This one is non-negotiable. In many areas it's a law that you can't be on your phone while driving.[9] Even in the areas where it's legal, it's still stupid. (But you're going to do it anyway.)

9 At the time of this writing distracted driving is illegal (and ticketable) in 47 states, D.C., Puerto Rico, Guam, and the US Virgin Islands.

You're six times more likely to cause an accident when you're on your phone than if you were driving drunk.[10] Listen, you could die. You could kill an innocent person—like yourself. (But you're going to do it anyway.) According to StopTextsStopWrecks.org, in the US in 2016, 3,450 people were killed in motor vehicle crashes involving distracted drivers. That's almost ten percent of all motor vehicle fatalities and it's getting worse. (But you're going to do it anyway.) No text message is that important. It can wait.

Speaking of waiting, I've saved one of my best behavior-changing tactics for this important moment. It's incredibly simple, but incredibly powerful. Even though none of the above (fines, lifelong guilt, or even death) will stop you, this will. You'll want to use this every time you want stop any bad habit. It alone is worth ten times what you've paid for this book in time and money. Ready?

Saying "I don't text and drive" to yourself every time you're tempted to check or respond to something while you're driving is much more effective than "I can't text and drive." That's it. One word. Science agrees that changing a single word matters. A *lot.* One study[11] found that sixty-four percent of people saying "I don't eat candy" were able to refuse a chocolate bar and only thirty-nine percent of people saying "I can't eat candy" could refuse it. In another, eight out of ten women who said "I don't skip workouts" kept up with their routine, but only ONE out of ten women who said "I can't skip workouts" stayed the course. "Cannot" happens to you, but "do not" happens because of you. "Do not" language is far more empowering.

---

10 *https://www.edgarsnyder.com/car-accident/cause-of-accident/cell-phone/cell-phone-statistics.html*

11 Patrick, V., & Hagtvedt, H. (2012). "I Don't" versus "I Can't": When Empowered Refusal Motivates Goal-Directed Behavior. *Journal of Consumer Research, 39*(2), 371-381. doi:10.1086/663212

If you "do not" check your phone while driving, then you might as well change your phone's settings to reflect that. Many phones offer a "driving mode" setting. Your phone will determine when you're driving and send an automated response to anyone who tries to reach you. If it's urgent, they can get the message to you right away. If it's not, then you'll get it when you arrive at your destination. I've used this for a long time and I can count on one hand the number of times a texter felt it was that important to reach me. Turn on your phone's driving mode right now.

Finally, make sure you don't cheat. Do whatever you have to do to avoid lying to your phone (and to yourself) by tapping the "I'm not driving" button. Make a promise. Make a vow. Sign a contract. (I've included one after this chapter.) Tell everyone who sits in your passenger seat to hold you accountable. Heck, lock the phone in the glove box so that you have to physically stop the car and take the key out of the ignition before you can get at your phone. Do whatever it takes—and then do some more. This is literally a life-or-death thing.

Meetings. Not quite as life-or-death as the previous no-phone-zone, but important nonetheless. We hear a lot about the challenge of building a strong corporate culture. We hear about generation gaps, in-fighting, cliques forming, cross-departmental bickering, low morale, high turnover, and on and on. The workplace is stressful, flawed, and we need to band together if we're going to do good work and enjoy the process.

Stephen Covey used a great analogy to teach about priorities. If you take a large jar and fill it with as many large rocks as you can, then it's still not full. You've got room for smaller rocks that can fall in between the spaces. And when you can't cram in any more smaller rocks, you can still pour some sand into the jar. Next, you'd be surprised by how much water you can pour into the jar without it overflowing.

Meetings are one example of how this can play out. The first thing many people do when they sit down for a meeting is pull out their phone and wait for the meeting to start. The phone will then get placed on the table momentarily until the meeting feels boring or irrelevant, only to be picked up again.

Simon Sinek reminds us that it's the tiny moments of face-to-face interaction that become the large rocks of relationship, connection, community, and ultimately, a positive culture. Unfortunately, the sand of phone time is pushing them out. There's no longer any space for one co-worker to say to the other, "Hey, how's your brother doing?"

Let meetings be a place where human connection can thrive. Let meetings be an environment where a group of people can focus on the issues and on each other. Let meetings be a no-phone-zone.

Phubbing. Phone snubbing is far too frequent a thing. A study in 2013[12] showed that just having a phone in sight during a conversation (even if it is face-down and off!) drastically reduces the quality of the interaction. When having a face-to-face conversation, just stick your phone in a pocket.

Dinner. For centuries, the dinner table has been a time for families to talk about their day and do some bonding. Holidays and

12 Andrew K. Przybylski and Netta Weinstein, "Can You Connect with Me Now? How the Presence of Mobile Communication Technology Influences Face-to-Face Conversation Quality," *Journal of Social and Personal Relationships* 30, no. 3 (May 2013): 237-46.

milestones are often celebrated with a special meal. The practice of Christianity has an ancient tradition of dining together that is appropriately called "Communion". There is just something about eating together that brings people together.

Phones have infiltrated our dinner tables and are often part of a place setting, sitting right alongside a knife and fork. In addition to dinner, you might want to consider establishing all meals as no-phone-zones in your household.

Tech Sabbath. Many people have found it helpful to pick one or more days per week to go completely device-free. Some religions require it, but even non-religious folks are picking up the practice. You can block off any days to do this, as long as you can stay consistent with it. 100% compliance is simpler and easier for your brain than 99%.

Tech Sunset. Same idea as a tech sabbath, but instead of a full-day, it's a period of time each and every evening when you go device-free. Roughly thirty minutes before bed until roughly thirty minutes after you wake up is a good place to start.

Kids. Parents will have to set and enforce no-phone-zones for their kids. For example, don't let them be on their phones alone in their room. Limit their daily screen time. Monitor what they're doing online. Keep infants under a year old away from phones and tablets altogether and "wait 'til eight!" (Don't allow your child their own device until they turn eight years of age.) For more, see the chapter titled, "An Extra Special Chapter For Parents."

Focus. You may want to start carving out time for activities that require deep focus. Focus is becoming rare indeed. Important things require focus. Reading, meditating, deep conversation, praying, studying, daydreaming, and solitude are all examples. Our attentions have become scattered. We skim, we scan, and we skip to the "TL/DR" summary (too long, didn't read.) Maybe it wasn't too long, maybe your attention span was too short. Focus is a skill that is lost without use. Without focus, we are without creativity, empathy, or self-identity. Knowledge becomes chunks of random information unattached to a context or overall narrative and meaningful productivity turns into frantically checking strings of items off a never-ending to-do list.

These are simply guidelines and suggestions. You are of course free to claim any date, time, place, situation, or emotion as a no-phone-zone. The point is to proactively set your own limits. Take a moment right now to decide which of the above suggestions you're going to implement. Then take the rest of the day to notice areas of your own life where your phone has become an unwelcome guest. Consider establishing a no-phone-zone for that in the future.

After completing Day Seven's "phast" you might also discover some more areas where you'll want to remove your phone on a more permanent basis.

Overwhelmed? It's important to realize that you're only making a list today. I recommend implementing no-phone-zones into your life one or two at a time. You might start with driving and maybe dinner and then add more as you see fit. If you forbid phones from ninety percent of your life all at once, then you're more likely to slip up. You want to build up a series of small wins, not set yourself up to fail.

CHAPTER CHECKLIST

- Have you made a list of no-phone-zones that you wish to establish?
- During the day, have you noticed areas and/or times that might make for a good no-phone-zone?
- Have you chosen which of your no-phone-zones you will establish first?
- Do you have a specific plan and time frame for establishing the rest?
- Have you signed the "no texting and driving" contract in the next chapter?
- Does your phone have "do not disturb" settings that automatically turn on while you're driving? Have you activated them?
- Have you changed your language from "I can't use my phone in no-phone-zones" to the more empowering, "I *do not* use my phone in no-phone-zones"?
- Have you noticed any improvements in your tracking app yet?
- Have you toasted your favorite beverage to your amazing progress so far?

THE DON'T TEXT AND DRIVE PLEDGE

Adapted from ItCanWait.com

According to the Virginia Tech Transportation Institute, those who text while driving are *23 TIMES* more likely to be in a crash.

I AM COMMITTED TO MAKING THE ROADS SAFER BY FOLLOWING THESE TIPS:

- **Be Smart.** Don't text and drive. No text message is worth a life.
- **Be Caring.** Don't send a text to a family member, friend, or co-worker when you know they're driving.
- **Be In Control.** Remember, it's your phone. You decide if and when to send and read texts so take control.

- **Be an Example.** A survey done by AT&T found that 77 percent of teens say adults tell them not to text and drive yet do it themselves "all the time." Still, 89 percent of those teens said their own parents are good role models in terms of not texting while driving. It's not just about you anymore.

I, ____
don't text and drive. No matter what the message is…it can wait.

DAY SIX: THE PLAY DATE

To this point, I've used words like "challenge," "contract," and "organize." You know what? It's time for a reward.

ACTION STEP: Make plans to get together with someone you haven't seen in a while.

That's it. Just plan to get together with someone you enjoy hanging out with, but you haven't had a chance to do so in a long time. I don't care what you do or for how long. Actually, that's not entirely true. The only rule is that this must be done in person! A Skype hangout won't cut it. Facetime isn't going to replace face-to-face time. A Zoom Meeting? You really need to find some friends outside of work.

You don't have to get together with them today, although you can, I just want you to make the firm plans by the end of the day today. Make it your singular mission and focus. The first person you reach out to may not reply right away. They may be on vacation. Heck, they may not want to see you. Reach out to someone else. You may have to reach out to five or ten people before you can get something on the calendar.

Do you feel awkward reaching out to someone you haven't spoken to in forever? Do it anyway. Blame it on me if you want. Tell them you're doing a "smart phoning challenge," and that you're using it as an excuse to do something you've been meaning to do for a while anyway. Or just be a normal human and say, "I miss your face. Life has been crazy, but we should totally get together soon. Would you be up for coffee next week? I'd love to catch up."

Important side note: When you do go somewhere with this person, leave your phone in the car. "But what if there's an emergency?" you ask. Don't worry. They'll have their phone on them.

CHAPTER CHECKLIST

- Have you made plans to get together, in person, face-to-face, with at least one real-live human that you haven't seen in a while?
- Have you indulged in a fond memory today?

DAY SIX: DO THIS FOR EXTRA CREDIT...

Everyone makes to-do lists. They're helpful for keeping us focused and on track.

But what if they are focusing us on the *wrong things?*

When I think about to-do lists, I think about "TASKS"—stuff that needs to get done—things that I can put a big red line through and mark as "completed." It feels like a productive day if I'm hunched over my computer, clearing out my inbox, editingn my latest book, and banging out projects one after the other.

But won't there be another list tomorrow?

> I once overheard a sobering comment, *"When you die, there will still be emails in your inbox."*

I regularly speak to audiences at conferences and events around the country and I talk about the magic of human connection. Through stories, science, humor, and a little magic, I help the event participants to stop and consider the value of developing and maintaining deep, meaningful relationships—even (and perhaps ESPECIALLY) in our modern digital world.

NOBODY has ever come up to me after my talk to argue that tasks are more important than relationships.

EVERYONE pays lip service to the fact that people are important and a top priority.

And then their phone dings and they get sucked right back into being "too busy."

Let's not be THAT person.

The problem with how people try to be productive is that they're too focused on accomplishing tasks, but the real way to have a productive day, is to create daily opportunities to nurture relationships. Instead of only writing out a to-do list, try adding a to-who list.

INSTEAD OF A LIST OF TASKS, A "TO-WHO" LIST IS A LIST OF NAMES.

- Who do you need to check in with today?
- Who do you need to thank?
- What relationship do you need to make a positive deposit into?
- Who could use a random act of kindness?
- Who haven't you seen in a while that you could do brunch with this week?

Write down four or five names and then follow through.

I get it. Dropping someone a note "just to say hi" doesn't feel very productive. But that's the thing about relationships. You can't mass-produce them. They don't scale. They each require their own special kind of manual labor to maintain.

And you will never be able to check them off as "completed."

But it's little things like doing a to-who list that make the difference between SAYING that you value these people and actually VALUING them.

TAKE THE 15-DAY "TO-WHO LIST" CHALLENGE

I challenge you to try writing a to-who list every weekday for three weeks.

Each time you write a to-do list, also write a "to-who" list. Some names can repeat, or you can come up with new names every time. Scroll through your social media connections if you need ideas for who to reach out to. You've already got the seeds of human connection in place. Now it's time to throw some water on them.

You'd have to do some mental gymnastics to imagine anything BAD coming from this. But it isn't difficult to see how this challenge could pay off for you in a big way. Nurtured relationships bear the best kind of fruit that life has to offer.

Why not start right now? Make a to-who list and start nurturing those relationships.

ACTION STEP: Make a To-WHO List Every Day for Three Weeks

DAY SEVEN: "PHAST"

ACTION STEP: Turn your phone off for 24 hours.

BREATHE.

DAY...EIGHT?

You've finished the seven-day challenge. Congratulations! Take some time today to evaluate your experience. Have a look at your tracking app. Was there any improvement from when you started? How do you feel? What have you learned? Have you made progress toward your target? Did the challenge "work" for you? How do you know?

Think about what happens next. Will you need to do the challenge again? Change it around a bit? Take it more (or less) seriously next time? Invite some different people along? Who are you going to challenge next?

I invited my first group of challenge participants to hop on a call and think through some of those questions with me. Nathan McGlothlin was one reader whose comments stuck out to me. He said, "These aren't just action steps. It's not that I'm going to just do it once and be done. These are practices. There's no reason why I shouldn't be able to reorganize my apps on a regular basis or change my lock screen again. That's just smart."

He's right. Your relationship with your phone is just that—a relationship. This challenge was a fun way to get you interacting with your phone differently, but it isn't the be all and end all solution. This is something that should be an ongoing process. Fortunately, I have a secret for you. During the challenge, you've learned new principles and concepts, you've developed new skills, and you've identified your priorities. These will all serve you well as you continue to design and live out your ideal relationship with technology.

Nathan is a busy guy. He's the Chief Experience Officer for a large university. That means he's got events to orchestrate, trainings to deliver, destinations to travel to, meetings to attend, and pop-ins galore. Spend ten minutes with him on campus and you'll quickly see that he is a go-to guy. Everyone has questions for Nathan and it's obvious why. Because regardless of your rank or standing in the organization, Nathan has an answer and a smile for you. Digitally, things are no different. Emails and texts are like virtual pop-ins that would threaten to kill anyone's productivity. But Nathan did it. He passed the seven-day challenge with flying colors. And he's just getting started. The day I spoke to him was his twenty-eighth day in a row staying under his goals for both time spent on his phone and number of unlocks. Not only that, but he's also invited others to do the challenge with him. They've agreed because heck, if someone as busy as Nathan can do it, then anyone can.

I'd love to hear from you. What was your individual experience? What sort of results did you get? What advice would you have for someone who is about to start their own seven-day challenge? I will personally read anything you send to tim@7daydigitaldiet.com.

WHAT IF IT DIDN'T WORK?

Desperate times call for desperate measures.

After completing your seven-day challenge you may still have some difficulties as your old phone habits begin to creep back into your life. Don't lose hope. There are still more techniques you can try. Some of them in this chapter are a bit goofy or even downright desperate, but every once in a while, even a wild Hail Mary pass is caught for a touchdown. You'll never know it until you throw it.

Remember the habit loop we learned about on Day One of the challenge? (Refresher: every habit is comprised of a cue, a routine, and a reward.) Your best shot for taming a bad smartphone habit is to replace the routine of swiping and staring with a new, healthy routine that moves you closer to your target and gratifies your brain's need for the same type of reward that checking your phone gives you. That was the focus of the seven-day challenge—identifying your highest values and feeding them instead of feeding your impulses.

But you can also have some success by tinkering with the other two pieces of the habit loop. You can remove the cues and you can dampen the reward that the unwanted behavior brings you. You could even turn what used to be a reward into a punishment. What follows is a buffet of ideas for attacking the habit loop at both the cue and the reward stages.

BREAK THE CUE

People who do a "digital detox," delete all their social media accounts, or drop their phone into a sewer drain are attempting to destroy the cues that cause their unwanted habits. There are two problems with this approach. First, it is insufficient. The brain will still crave the reward and seek out a suitable gratifying behavior. Typically, these people just end up starting another bad habit instead. Second, it is impractical. An alcoholic might be able to keep alcohol out of the house, but you cannot extract technology from your life as you know it. There are of course the options of moving to a monastery, a convent, or to Amish Country, but for most of us, these are not really options.

But it doesn't hurt to reduce cues where possible as long as you're doing so in conjunction with your work on the rest of the habit loop. Here are some ideas to remove or minimize cues.

1. Throw tire spikes in front of your problem apps.

Part of the reason smartphones become a problem for some people is they are quick and easy to operate. Do you remember when slot machines took actual quarters? And they had this big arm you had to crank to set the wheels spinning? Now all you have to do is push a little button and your credits (not called money) automatically drain from your account. It's MUCH easier. Instead of one game per spin, video slots now present you with this complex grid of fifteen different lines. It's MUCH faster. Your brain loves it when routine behaviors are quick and easy. So, you're going to make using some of your apps slow and painful.

If there is an app you find yourself coming back to again and again, then you might consider it a problem app. I had a certain game that ate up way too much of my time, but I couldn't seem to shake it. I once did a thirty-day, no video game challenge and I successfully abstained from all games, including this one. In fact, I never went back to any of the others. Cold turkey worked for those games, but the moment the thirty days was up, I found myself drawn back in to this one problem app. I had to try something else. Here's what I've found works for me now.

I don't just close the app when I'm done playing. I delete it. Every time. If I want to play it again, I'm forced to reinstall. I mean, the game is fun, but it's not *that* fun. If changing your lock screen is like installing a speed bump, then this is like throwing down tire spikes. The cue is still there, but it takes just long enough between cue and routine, that I often catch myself beforehand.

2. Bombard your future self.

Write out your target and/or your reasons why you want to reach it on some sticky notes and put them where you'll see them. On your bathroom mirror, at your work station, on your computer, in your wallet, and as a bookmark are all good suggestions. The idea is to do everything you can to get the message through to your stubborn, habit-driven, subconscious mind. Seeing positive encouragement everywhere will help to crowd out any negative cues from showing up.

3. Use this magic phrase.

One of the cues for pulling out your phone is when someone else pulls out theirs. It isn't pleasant when you're with someone who is just staring at their phone. But it isn't always polite or appropriate to tell them what to do either. The approach I've found that works best is simply asking, "Is everything okay?" It's a gentle, caring reminder that you are both in this room, at this moment, together. Most of the time, they'll get the hint, get off their phone, and explain briefly what they were doing. Sometimes though, everything is not okay. I was doing a leadership training for a small company and somebody in the room was on her phone to the point of distraction. I stopped and politely asked, "Is everything okay?"

"No," she said. "My nephew from Oregon was in a major car accident this morning and now we don't know if he's even going to make it."

Can you imagine if I just pulled out my phone and distanced myself at the exact moment another human being needed some empathy? Or worse, can you imagine if I had barked at her with some self-important demand for attention?

One of the things emphasized throughout this book is the fact that phones aren't all bad. You should be able to intentionally use your phone as often as you truly want to. Knowing that, isn't it also true that we should give others permission to intentionally use theirs? We don't jump to the extreme ideas until we know that the simple ones won't work.

4. Put Dorothy back into her house.

In *The Wizard of Oz*, a tornado blew Dorothy and her house right out of that boring sepia-toned world and straight into Technicolor.

And you have to admit, Oz is an incredible place. It's much better than Kansas. I'm not even going to apologize to Kansas here. It's so obviously true.

Here's your goal: make your phone more like Kansas. We know that phone designers want their phones to be more like Oz. They want the bright colors to be a cue that pulls us in. But there's no place like home. Real life should feel more like Oz and your phone should feel more like Kansas. Unfortunately to many, it's the other way around. It isn't just the wonder and enchantment of a new world that our phones give us access to. It's also the look and feel that draws us in. Our phones are bright, colorful, delightfully noisy objects. It's no wonder our brains find them so appealing. We're going to change that by reducing your phone's default brightness, going grayscale, and killing every last beep, ding, and whistle.

Step-by-step tutorials for all three can be found at www.7DayDigitalDiet.com/resources. Grayscale will take some getting used to, so I'll teach you a hack for using your home button to toggle back and forth between grayscale and color. Then you'll be able to cyclone in and out of Kansas whenever you want.

5. Be a social drinker.

Don't you hate it when you're out to eat and the person you're with only has eyes for their phone? There is a bar in Brazil that has solved this problem. They serve their beer in glasses that will only stand upright if perched on top of a cell phone. For a picture, visit: www.7DayDigitalDiet.com/fun. That's the weirdest/awesomest drinking game I've ever heard of. There might be cues present to check your phone, but you simply can't unless you want to take a drink (or spill a drink.)

6. Take a power nap.

We lost power in our house for three days once. By the second night we were having so much fun playing board games by candlelight that I secretly wished the power would never come back on. So now, about twice a year I sneak downstairs to flip the circuit breaker. Then, I pretend to be annoyed at the "inconvenience" while I break out the Yankee candles and Monopoly board. We might not be able to remove technology from our lives completely, but we can certainly give ourselves a break now and then.

7. Get yourself a signal-blocking "focus sleeve."

Sometimes you only want to temporarily eliminate cues. One option is to simply set your phone to airplane mode or turn it off entirely for a predetermined period while you focus on something else. Another is to use a signal-blocker. A signal-blocker is a small pouch that keeps all cell, Bluetooth, and WiFi signals out. While your phone is inside, it will be unable to transmit or receive in any manner.

DAMPEN THE REWARD

The idea now is to take the reward that your brain is accustomed to feeling while on your phone and make it *less* rewarding. If the reward isn't so great, then perhaps you won't be so compelled to complete the behavior. The higher a drug gets you, the more addictive it is. Diminish the high and you diminish its addictive pull.

1. Engage the Demetricator.

This sounds like a super-villain's tool of destruction, but in truth, it is a browser plug-in battling for the forces of good.

Facebook and the "Like" button seem as though they've always been together. Like bread and butter, peanut butter and jelly, or Flavor Flav and clocks. But for Facebook's first five years, social media's premier pioneering platform existed without its most iconic feature. It is even reported that Facebook founder, Mark Zuckerberg turned down the idea of a like button (dubbed the "awesome button" at the time) because he felt it would pull users away from more engaging activities such as commenting and sharing.

As it turns out, posts that are "Liked" move up users' feeds and are viewed by more people, more often, and end up garnering *more* comments and shares—not less. Impressive, but that's not how the Like button revolutionized social media. That innocent-looking thumbs up icon (and the all-important number next to it) scratches one of your deepest and most pervasive psychological itches—the need for social approval. When lots of people like your post or photo, dopamine levels spike in your brain to just below where they would be if you had snorted cocaine or won the jackpot. That's a very desirable reward. It's no wonder we find ourselves compulsively checking our social media sites at the first whiff of a free moment. It's no wonder Facebook users collectively post an average of 510,000 comments, 293,000 status updates, and 136,000 photos per *minute*. We're looking for our next feel-good hit of social acceptance. If you multiply that by Twitter, Instagram, SnapChat, YouTube, LinkedIn, and virtually every other successful social media platform out there, then it's no wonder why people have grown to conflate quantity of connection with quality. Enter the Demetricator.

Benjamin Grosser noticed his own growing obsession with peer approval. On his web site, he describes how he knew it had gotten out of hand. "How many likes did my photos get today? What's my friend count? How much did people like my status? I focused on these quantifications, watching for the counts of responses rather than the responses themselves, or waiting for numbers of friend requests to appear rather than looking for meaningful connections." That's why he created the Facebook Demetricator. "The Facebook interface is filled with numbers," he explains. "These numbers, or metrics, measure and present our social value and activity, enumerating friends, likes, comments, and more. Facebook Demetricator is a web browser add-on that hides these metrics. Friend counts disappear. '16 people like this' becomes 'people like this'." Those who use it report being less focused on how many friends they have or on how much people like their statuses, and more focused on who they are and what they said. The Demetricator (available for Twitter and Instagram as well) attempts to dampen the intensity of the reward that quantity brings.

2. Fool your hands.

What if your brain's reward is simply the satisfying and reassuring feel of a phone in your hands? I've heard of at least two products that simulate the look and feel of a smartphone, but they contain no digital features. One, called "Realism," is simply a glass frame in the size and shape of your standard smartphone. Hold it up and look through it if you want, but all you'll see is the real world on the other side. The other is the "Substitute Phone," which was inspired by a documentary about a man who quit smoking by replacing his pipe with a stick. The Substitute Phone is a rectangular piece of heavy black plastic with a row of round beads embedded across its face. Rolling your thumb over the beads mimics the action of swiping a phone and may be enough of a reward to keep your real phone hidden away in your pocket. (You can see a video of the Substitute Phone in action at www.7DayDigitalDiet.com/fun.)

PUT MUSTARD ON YOUR NIPPLE

I remember the time a new baby arrived in our neighborhood. I wasn't much more than a toddler myself and our moms were close, so the four of us ended up spending a lot of time together. I didn't speak much as a kid, so people spoke freely in front of me.

"How's the baby doing with the bottle? Any luck?"

"No, I can't get him to give up the breast."

"Did you try putting a little bit of mustard on your nipple? One taste and he'll never want to nurse again!"

Instead of reducing your brain's reward, we're going to go in the other direction. We're going to look at ways that you can punish your brain whenever you're caught in the act. Your brain is like a pet or a child that needs to be trained. There's nothing like a good old stick when the carrot fails. There's nothing like the rude awakening of a bitter taste when you're expecting something sweet. The following ideas may shock your system. That's the point.

1. Get blasted.

The concept is quite simple. Give an airhorn to your closest friend or spouse and have them blast it every time they catch you phubbing them. ("Phubbing" is short for "phone snubbing"—the act of ignoring someone else in favor of your phone.) You'll find a video of a guy doing this to his girlfriend repeatedly at www.7DayDigitalDiet.com/fun. The video looks scripted and the acting is bad, but I think we can assume that her anger response is close enough to what would happen in real life. Don't do it to anyone unless they've asked you to. That way, nobody will get mad. Except maybe the neighbors.

2. Pull a Maneesh.

Maneesh Sethi claims he once hired a girl to slap him in the face every time she saw him wasting time on Facebook. Well, that's one way to do it. The other way is with Sethi's ensuing invention, Pavlok. You wear Pavlok on your wrist like a watch, it links to your phone and either buzzes, beeps, or gives you an electric shock whenever you are misusing your device. This is a flexible tool and can be used to break just about any bad habit. According to the web site, "Seventy-five percent of smokers (and eighty percent of nail-biters) who used Pavlok quit in as little as five days and were still free [of the offending habit] six months later." Physical pain too much for you? Let's try emotional pain.

3. Embarrass yourself.

Here's an idea. Buy an ugly phone. Your brain cares deeply about what other people think. I know, it's stupid. But it's biology. I recently smashed my sleek black phone and needed to buy a new one that day. The only color anyone had in stock was "rose gold." (That's a euphemism for "shiny pink.") When you own an ugly phone (or in my case, a phone that's a little *too* pretty), you'll be surprised at how mortified you'll be to bring it out any time there are people around. Public embarrassment is something that feels like it needs to be avoided at all costs. You can use this as powerful motivation to keep your phone in your pocket when there are other people around (which is exactly when your phone *should* be in your pocket.)

If you don't want to waste all that money on an ugly phone, then try slapping on an ugly phone case or an ugly sticker instead. I understand that "ugly" is a relative term but use your imagination. Are you a forty-year-old business man? Then attach that Twilight Sparkle My Little Pony phone case to your Blackberry so tightly that you'd need power tools to get it off. Harry Potter fan and die-hard Ravenclaw? Then pick out a case bearing the green crest of Slytherin. Vegan? Then put a sticker on the back of your phone that says, "I LOVE BACON!" Don't bother with subtlety here. Enlist the help of your closest friends, if you must. I'm sure they'll have great ideas for ways that you can counteract your own politics, heckle your own religion, and/or defile your own beliefs. Trust me. They've been wanting to do this for years.

4. Fine!?

Maybe physical and emotional pain have no effect on you. Let's try kicking you straight in the wallet. Get a jar and label it, "The Phub Bucket." Any time you phub someone close to you, drop a predetermined fine into the jar. When it is full, use the money to go somewhere fun together. What do you think, good idea?

Uri Gneezy and Aldo Rustichini wanted to challenge the assumption that issuing a monetary penalty discourages unwanted behavior. They conducted a famous experiment that involved charging parents a fine for picking up their kids late from day care. As it turns out, fining people doesn't work to decrease unwanted behavior, it actually INCREASES it instead!

"Parents used to arrive late to collect their children, forcing a teacher to stay after closing time. We introduced a monetary fine for late-coming parents. As a result, the number of late-coming parents increased significantly."[13]

Phubbing becomes okay in your mind because you've paid for it. It's a transactional solution instead of a relational solution. Worse yet, it all ends with a *reward* of doing something fun. Let's try a more sinister mind game on yourself. Something that has proven to be effective instead of counter-productive.

5. Support the Ku-Klux Klan.

"WHAT!?" you exclaim. "That is outrageous! I would NEVER support the KKK!"

Okay, okay. Then donate to the Nazis instead.

This idea involves choosing a cause that you absolutely despise and giving them money every time you break your promise to yourself. The cause must be utterly unworthy of your money if this is going to work.

Maybe it's an organization that is notoriously cruel to animals. Maybe it's a company or political candidate you vehemently disagree with. Maybe it's a person you hate. Write them a check and give it to a trusted friend to hold. If you are caught in a bad habit loop, then your friend is instructed to mail it off.

Don't have a friend you can trust? StickK.com is a web site that will take on that role for you. If you're ready to put your phone in its place, then maybe it's time to put your money where your mouth is. Besides, the real hope here is that you won't have to mail any checks at all.

---

13 *https://papers.ssrn.com/sol3/papers.cfm?abstract_id=180117*

If you do want to donate to a worthy cause, I recommend an organization such as the Center for Humane Technology. Their mission is to (strongly) encourage developers to design their products with our values in mind and not just the dollar value of our attention. It's a worthy cause and a capable crew. Donate to the Center for Humane Technology here: https://humanetech.com/donate/

Got any creative ideas to share? I'd love to put them in the next edition of this book along with your name! What are you doing to keep your phone habits in check? Email your ideas over to me at: tim@7DayDigitalDiet.com.

AN EXTRA SPECIAL CHAPTER FOR PARENTS

Okay, fellow parents. It's time we had a chat. The average young person spends an average of a lot of hours per day staring at a screen. A *LOT*. Depending on the source, I've seen it placed anywhere from one hour and fifty-five minutes per day, to almost nine hours per day. Accounting for the time spent in school and sleeping, that's almost every waking moment. But did you really need research to tell you that your kids are spending a lot of time staring at screens? You've probably noticed it yourself, right?

Here's what you may not have noticed: at least *some* of that is our fault as their parents. That's *good* news. It means that what we do makes a difference. We have the ability (and responsibility) to help our kids figure out—and live out—a healthy relationship with their phones. Surprise! This chapter is really about you.

I once read a story about a man in China who realized that he had an influence over his adult son's relationship to technology. This father had the best of intentions, but maybe not exactly the best plan of action. He was so fed up with how much time his son was spending playing video games that he hired "digital hit men" in the form of other gamers to kill off all his son's characters. There was no word on whether it worked, no tips on where to find digital hit men, how much they charge, (or even how to apply for a job like that.) Even if it was successful in improving his son's relationship to tech, I'm sure it wasn't so great for improving his son's relationship to his father. Your goal is to be a loving parent, not a heartless tyrannical dictator.

"Loving parent" doesn't mean "let your kids do whatever they want." I get it. We're all busy. Tossing a phone to a kid is a pretty darn effective way to keep THEM busy (and keep them quiet.) I do see the appeal. On the one hand, we know that excessive screen time for our kids is unhealthy. On the other hand, we know that technology isn't going anywhere, and we want our kids to keep up in a competitive world. On the other hand, it would be nice to have more face-to-face time with our kids. On the other hand, it would be nice if they would just stay still and quiet for ten minutes. Parenting today has some new and unique challenges that the world has never seen before. How are we going to pull this off?

Frankly, it starts with leading by example. Like it or not, our kids will mimic us for better or for worse. Newborn babies gravitate toward smartphones not only because of the bright colors, but also because they see everyone else around them staring at a similar device. We complain about how much time our kids spend on their phones, but what about us? Are we being hypocrites? You can't hand this book over to your kids and expect it to "fix" them unless you're willing to rise to the challenge yourself.

They may not say anything to you, but your kids do notice how often you're on your phone. Kindergarten kids in Boston were asked to imagine the best playground ever. They agreed that the best way to design a park was to have a locker to "lock up the parent's cell phones so they'll actually play with us." Only three percent of parents surveyed said they "strictly" limit their tech use around their kids. That leaves ninety-seven percent who are passive about what their kids see them doing. Here's what I know...

There's nothing more powerful
than your loving example.

Now, just because it's good for your kids to see you consistently following the rules, doesn't mean that you should have the *same exact rules* as them. You're an adult. The rules are almost always different for adults. Children's brains require different sets of phone usage boundaries than adult brains do. This is NOT a free pass for you to go crazy, it's just a fact.

Listen, your kids are going to need your help managing their own technology usage. It's just too much for them. Don't give a six-year-old a smartphone and say, "Now, try to limit your screen time, Little Johnny." That's like handing a teenage boy the keys to a brand-new Porsche, putting him on an open stretch of road, and telling him to go slow.

Here's what the top experts at the *American Academy of Pediatrics* recommend for your kids:

Less than Eighteen Months Old

Absolutely no screen time (with the exception of allowing some video chat time with Grandma.)

Between Eighteen Months and Five Years old

Allow less than an hour of high-quality children's programming per day.

Between Five Years Old and Seven Years Old

Set and enforce consistent limits and do not allow them to have their own device yet. (Just remember, "Wait 'till eight!")

Between Eight Years Old and the Early Teenage Years

Despite what your preteen, tween, and young teenage kids may think, you are still in charge. You can always change the WiFi password in your home. That password is a privilege, not a right. The same is true for their phone's unlock password. During this phase, you should have veto power over every one of your kids' phoning sessions. If they want to go on it, you'll have to enter the unlock code. When you do, I recommend immediately setting a timer ON THEIR PHONE for the length of time they are allowed to use it. When the timer goes off, they must stop whatever they are doing and return the phone to you. (HINT FROM EXPERIENCE: Set your own timer as well. Otherwise, they'll try to stretch it out.) Don't forget any no-phone-zones that you set on Day Six of the challenge. In addition to those, I recommend adding one more—your child's bedroom. They should not be permitted to use their smartphone in their own bedroom with their door closed. That's just a safety issue. As always, the key here is to set and adhere to consistent limits.

Beyond

At this stage of the game, you simply aren't in control of your kids' behavior the same way that you were when they were younger. Their independence is growing and so is their rebelliousness. Despite this, you are still a heavy influence in your child's life. Your best bet is to talk to them. Ask your kids if they know what phone manufacturers and software developers are trying to do to them. Ask them who the technology companies really want to help. Ask them what they want from life and whether or not their phones are helping them to get it. Ask lots of questions and *listen* to what they tell you. And of course, lead by example.

> "'Take care of yourself online OR ELSE' is wildly ineffective for teens because teens are not entirely in control of what is posted about them. 'Take care of one another,' is better." - Dr. Carrie James, research associate and lecturer at Harvard School of Education

One of the greatest gifts you can give anyone is your full attention. You don't have to be perfect, just present. Make eye contact. Listen actively. Make them feel heard, valued, and understood. Our culture is quickly becoming one of fragmented, shortened, and shallow attention. Make sure your child has the regular experience of being seen. Deprive them of food for a while if you have to, but don't deprive them of you.

As far as specific tactics and techniques for helping them to use their phones less, see the rest of this book. Take your child through the seven-day challenge or better yet, do it together as a family. It will work if you work it. Consistency is key and therefore worth repeating. Be aware as new technologies make their way into your child's home, school, and social circles. Notice how your children are affected by them and work hard to replace any deficiencies you see. For example, if you notice your child's attention span has been shortened, then foster in them a love of reading, prayer/meditation, thoughtful conversation, or any other focus-boosting activity. It's not really about using our phones less. It's about getting more out of life. It's about developing the skills, perspectives, and relationships that make life simpler and more fulfilling.

For a list of resources, ideas, web sites—and even inspiration—visit www.7DayDigitalDiet.com/parents. You're not alone in this.

WHAT YOU CAN DO TO HELP

I wrote this book to help people who want to phone less and live more. My humble hope is that it makes a genuine difference in how people relate to their devices. But sometimes I feel like I'm fighting a losing battle. I look around at everyone's faces illuminated by pale blue screens and I worry there aren't enough people who see the value in looking up every once in a while. Every time someone tells me to "just relax," accuses me of being a Luddite, or says that "everyone else has that problem but not me," I question if all the effort is worth it. I wonder if I should just focus on my own relationship with technology and my kids' relationship with technology and leave it at that.

But then I hear stories from the people who were helped by this challenge. I think about the wife who walked her husband through the challenge and told me it brought them closer together. I think about the kid who was given an earlier version of this book as a random gift. He reluctantly read it, did the challenge, and sent me a heartfelt thank-you email telling me how he climbed a mountain and how reaching the top felt like a turning point in his life. That's the kind of stuff that reminds me that it *is* worth it. That's what makes me want to do more. But these are just small ripples in a big pond. If we're going to make any kind of significant headway, then we're going to need to start making waves.

I can't make waves without you. Period. Word-of-mouth is at the core of every movement and there are several small things you can do that will make a BIG difference. There's also one BIG thing you can do, but I'll save the best for last.

1. Leave an online book review

This might be the single biggest thing you could do to raise awareness about this book and by extension, its message. I would consider it a personal favor. Reviews from readers are a HUGE part of what gets a book noticed today. Reviews help shoppers to make better decisions, retailers to sell more books, and authors to get their message out. Just to put the power of an individual reader's book review in perspective, The *New York Times* did a review of one of my books. It was nice, but I'd rather have an honest review from you. Not only is your review going to last longer, but it will have more influence on what real readers are going to decide to read next.

Here's the link with simple instructions (and links) for posting reviews on sites like Amazon and GoodReads: www.7DayDigitalDiet.com/review

I hate that I have to specify *honest* but unfortunately, fake reviews are becoming a real problem. So please use the link above to post your **HONEST** review(s) of this book. It's perfectly acceptable to copy and paste your review to multiple web sites.

Oh, and before you do anything...*thank you.* My gratitude for each and every review cannot be overstated. Yes, I do still read them all. And yes, I do still get giddy with excitement over every one.

2. Share on social media (I share back!)

I LOVE seeing posts about my book on social media. Besides the obvious benefit of reaching more people with this message, it's another way for me to connect with my readers. Writing can be a lonely gig. I want to know you're out there.

When you post something, PLEASE—for the love of all that is social—TAG ME! I will very likely comment, like, re-post, re-tweet, or forward your post to the rest of my readership.

Below, I've listed my current social media accounts. I'm not everywhere, and I'm not on all the time (obviously), but these are my active accounts:

- Facebook – www.fb.me/timdavidspeaks
- LinkedIn – www.linkedin.com/in/timdavidmagic
- Twitter – www.twitter.com/timdavidmagic
- Instagram – www.instagram.com/timdavidmagic

Remember, continue to use social media responsibly!

3. Suggest the challenge to a group that you belong to.

Is there a small group that you belong to? Would you consider suggesting that they go through the seven-day challenge together? Are you part of a work team? Bring it up at a meeting and point out that it will help everyone to be more connected, focused, and productive. Perhaps there is even a digital wellness program at your organization that this challenge could be added to as part of the curriculum. Are you a member of a civic group or community group? After you do the challenge internally, perhaps you could roll it out to the community? Are you in a support group? Share how changing your phone habits have helped you take control in other areas of your life too. Tell your networking group how this challenge has allowed you to form better connections with those around you. Are you in a book club? What do you know? This is a book! Any group works—even if it's just your group of friends or your own family.

When talking about this to people, remember that this is an *invite*, not a sale. You're *sharing* something, not pushing it. Relax. Just say that you did a cool thing and you want to know if they might enjoy doing the cool thing too.

4. Gift the book to someone.

Can you think of ONE person, right now who would appreciate a copy of this book? Give 'em a copy! You don't need a special occasion to give someone a gift. This is the most obvious and direct way that word-of-mouth works. People sharing stuff with each other.

That concludes my list of suggestions for SMALL actions that can lead to BIG results. Now it's time to turn these ripples into waves. I've saved the best for last…

5. Lead a group through the seven-day challenge.

For this to work, you need to be in a leadership position of some kind. I'm not only talking about a "boss" with "employees" in the traditional sense. Teachers can do this challenge with their students. (Side note for teachers reading this—I'm interested in putting together a downloadable Tech Wellness Curriculum of some kind. I have no idea where to begin doing that. I just know that this stuff needs to be taught in schools. Lil' help?) Coaches can lead their players through the challenge. Youth pastors can transform some of their kids' phone time into Bible time. Librarians can promote the challenge to their communities and encourage reading time over screen time. Parents can lead their families through the challenge. On and on it goes. Be creative. I know there are people in your life who you can help. Like Mark Sanborn says, "You don't need a title to be a leader."

Let me know how I can help you. I'm serious about this. Do you need bulk copies? Do you want me to create custom copies with your organization's logo and a special message inside? Do you just need some advice about getting started? Do you want me to come deliver a workshop for your group? Email me. Anything sent to tim@7DayDigitalDiet.com will come straight to my inbox and I'll personally read it.

Would you prefer to chat on the phone? Visit www.TimDavidPrepCall.com and pick out a time that works for you. Include a little note about what we'll be discussing, and I'll call you at the appropriate time. I'm not kidding. I will call you on the phone and we will talk one-on-one.

Pick one of the above suggestions and do it today, while you're thinking about it. Even if your small action only helps one person to turn one minute of phone time into one minute of quality time with a loved one, then it was significant and meaningful. THANK YOU, from the bottom of my heart.

If you're reading this because someone else did one of the above for you, then now would be a good time to personally thank them. Acknowledge the contribution they made, the effort they put in, or the money they invested in you. Let them know how their actions helped improve your life for the better. They didn't have to, but they did. Thank them.

ACKNOWLEDGEMENTS

I'm thankful for my phone.

Forgive the apparent irony. Today is March 21, 2020. It's the early stages of the Corona Virus pandemic. Everything is shut down and we're being strongly advised to stay home. Yet my devices have allowed me to stay productive in my work and connected to the people who matter to me. That was the whole point of a journey that ended up becoming this book. Despite the dangers of tech overuse, there are also downsides to tech *under*-use. So, I'm genuinely thankful for my phone, its developers, and the people who make it go.

That's a long list. Much shorter, is the list of individuals who stood up to voice an unpopular opinion in the midst of such an exciting technological revolution. Just like the poem at the beginning of this book, there are two sides to every truth. It takes a special mind to see the version of truth that is hidden. The following individuals have inspired me to think upstream: Sherry Turkle,

Adam Alter, Catherine Price, John T. Cacioppo and William Patrick, Alex and Brett Harris, Nicholas Kardaras, James P. Steyer, Nir Eyal, Charles Duhigg, and Brendan Burchard are just some of the giants whose shoulders I stand upon.

Thank you to anyone who has ever trusted me with an audience. I will never take for granted the gift of congregating with the sole purpose of sharing ideas, energy, and connection.

I'm increasingly thankful for my readers—or the case of this book—the doers. You've read advance copies, suffered through early attempts at the 7-day challenge, supported the Kickstarter campaign, given advice, brainstormed, shared results, and have been anything but passive consumers of the words I arrange.

Who are you thankful for?

ALSO BY TIM DAVID

It makes writing way more fun when there are readers out there, so ***thank you***. If you liked this, then you should know that I've also written two other books.

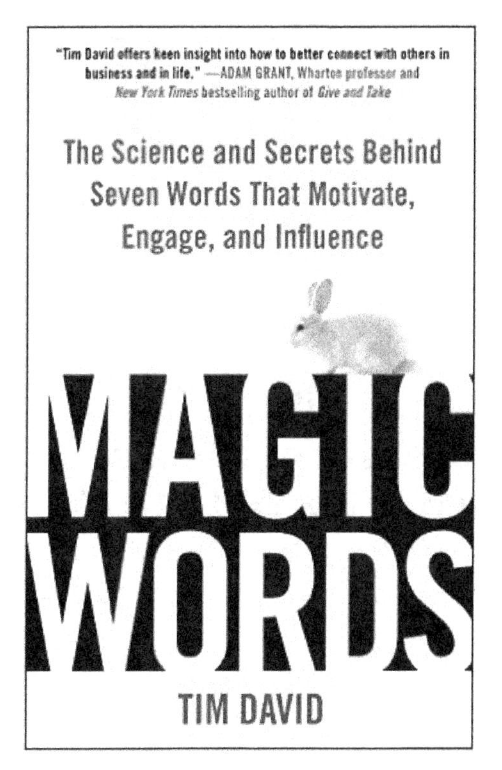

Magic Words: The Science and Secrets Behind Seven Words that Motivate, Engage, and Influence

Available in hardcover, ebook, and audiobook formats at: www.MagicWordsBook.com

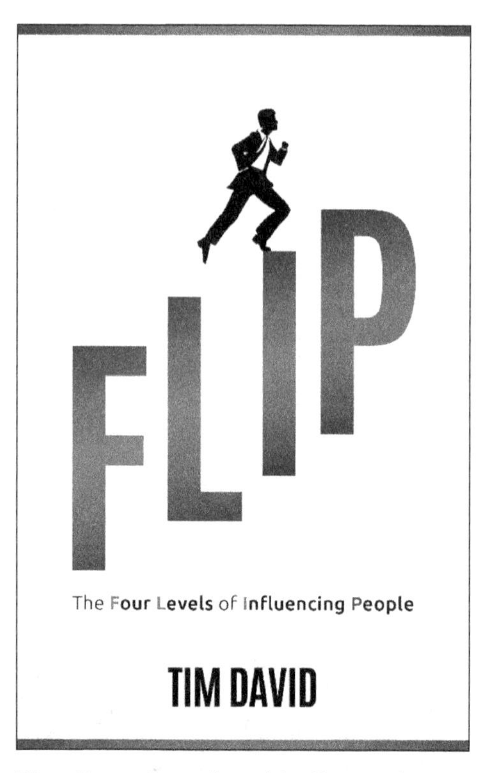

FLIP: The Four Levels of Influencing People

Available in paperback, ebook,
and audiobook formats at:
www.FlipTheBook.info

Or find them both (along with plenty of free resources for creating more human connection at work and in life) by visiting: www.GoodAtPeople.com

NOTES